Functions of Vitamins beyond Recommended Dietary Allowances

Bibliotheca Nutritio et Dieta

No. 55

Series Editors *P. Walter*, Basel
J.C. Somogyi, Rüschlikon-Zürich

KARGER
Basel · Freiburg · Paris · London · New York ·
New Delhi · Bangkok · Singapore · Tokyo · Sydney

Functions of Vitamins beyond Recommended Dietary Allowances

Volume Editors *P. Walter*, Basel
D. Hornig, Basel
U. Moser, Basel

34 figures and 26 tables, 2001

KARGER

Basel · Freiburg · Paris · London · New York ·
New Delhi · Bangkok · Singapore · Tokyo · Sydney

Paul Walter

Biochemisches Institut
Vesalianum, Universität Basel
Vesalgasse 1
CH–4051 Basel (Switzerland)

Ulrich K. Moser

F. Hoffmann-La Roche Ltd
Vitamins and Fine Chemicals Division
CH–4070 Basel (Switzerland)

Dietrich Hornig

F. Hoffmann-La Roche Ltd
Vitamins and Fine Chemicals Division
CH–4070 Basel (Switzerland)

Library of Congress Cataloging-in-Publication Data

European Academy of Nutritional Sciences. Workshop (1997 : Nice, France)
Functions of vitamins beyond recommended dietary allowances/
volume editors, P. Walter, D. Hornig, U. Moser.
p. ; cm. – (Bibliotheca nutritio et dieta; no. 55)
Includes bibliographical references and index.
ISBN 3805570732 (hard cover : alk. paper)
1. Vitamins in human nutrition – Congresses. I. Walter, Paul, 1933– . II. Hornig, D.H.
III. Moser, U. (Ulrich), 1946– . IV. Title. V. Series.
[DNLM: 1. Vitamins – physiology – Congresses. 2. Nutrition Policy – Congresses. QU
160 E89f 2001]
TX341.B5 no. 55
[QP771]
613.2′86–dc21 00–043435

Bibliographic Indices. This publication is listed in bibliographic services, including Current Contents® and Index Medicus.

Drug Dosage. The authors and the publisher have exerted every effort to ensure that drug selection and dosage set forth in this text are in accord with current recommendations and practice at the time of publication. However, in view of ongoing research, changes in government regulations, and the constant flow of information relating to drug therapy and drug reactions, the reader is urged to check the package insert for each drug for any change in indications and dosage and for added warnings and precautions. This is particularly important when the recommended agent is a new and/or infrequently employed drug.

www.karger.com
Printed in Switzerland on acid-free paper by Reinhardt Druck, Basel
ISSN 0067–8198
ISBN 3–8055–7073–2

Contents

Preface

More and more has become known on new properties and functions of various nutrients in our food. Of particular interest are functions of single or combinations of vitamins which seem to be involved in the improvement of immune function and in the risk reduction of chronic diseases such as cardiovascular diseases, cancer, and also neurological disorders like Alzheimer disease. The about 50 experts of the workshop that was held under the auspices of the European Academy of Nutritional Sciences in October 1997 discussed the progress in this area in great detail. In the summary discussions, which are also part of this book, the questions were raised for which of the vitamins recommendations can be formulated or if the necessary evidence is still missing and what the estimated time scale for obtaining this knowledge will be. Since not only scientists but also the consumers are very much interested in this development especially concerning the reduction of the risk of chronic diseases it was also discussed how the consumer should be informed on the progress science is making.

This volume of 'Bibliotheca Nutritio et Dieta' is the last one both under my editorship and the present name. Starting with No. 56, the series will change its name to 'Forum of Nutrition', with Professor I. Elmadfa from Vienna as the new editor and myself as co-editor.

Paul Walter

Walter P, Hornig D, Moser U (eds): Functions of Vitamins beyond Recommended Dietary Allowances. Bibl Nutr Dieta. Basel, Karger, 2001, No 55, pp 1–3

A Conceptual Approach for Scientifically Based Guidelines

P. Walter [a], *D. Hornig* [b], *U. Moser* [b]

[a] Swiss Vitamin Institute and Department of Biochemistry, University of Basel,
[b] F. Hoffmann-La Roche Ltd, Vitamins and Fine Chemicals Division, Basel, Switzerland

This book will review the scientific evidence for vitamin intake based on functions beyond the classical deficiencies. The objective is to elaborate guidelines for vitamin intake in individuals to cover new functions for these nutrients. Of particular interest are functions of single or of combinations of vitamins which may contribute to the prevention or risk reduction of chronic disease.

It is generally accepted that the basic needs of vitamins are covered by the intake equivalent to the Recommended Dietary Allowances (RDAs) which were originally established mainly to prevent deficiencies. RDAs are defined as 'the levels of intake of essential nutrients that, on the basis of scientific knowledge, are judged to be adequate to meet the known nutritional needs of practically all healthy persons'. What is meant by 'practically all healthy persons'? The individual requirements for each nutrient are conventionally assumed to have gaussian distribution. The RDA value is set as the mean requirement of the group plus 2 standard deviations, i.e. covering at least 97.5% of the population. RDAs are often misinterpreted because they are regarded as the lowest acceptable intake for each individual which is of course not true since most of the individuals may actually meet their requirements at a lower value. Furthermore, in most cases, RDAs include a factor relevant to each nutrient to account for the variation in turnover rates and body pools.

It is important to realize that even the more recently re-evaluated RDAs are still based essentially on the vitamin requirements to prevent the classical deficiencies (see for instance SCF report on 'Nutrient and Energy Intake for the European Community', 1992, and the report of the Department of Health (UK) on 'Dietary Reference Values for Food Energy and Nutrients for the United Kingdom', 1991). However, more and more scientific evidence is accumulating that several vitamins exhibit additional function each with a different requirement that is usually somewhat higher than the one for the prevention of the respective classical vitamin deficiency. Such functions include e.g. the radical scavenging effect of various antioxidant vitamins, the role of folate in the prevention of neural tube defect, and the effects of folate, vitamins B_6 and B_{12} in the regulation of the homocysteine concentration in blood. It is the goal of this workshop to substantiate the relations between the scientific evidence for selected functions and the respective vitamin intake.

Some functions apparently require not only one but several vitamins due to observed synergistic interactions. A typical example is the established synergism between the antioxidant vitamins C, E and β-carotene as radical scavengers. Therefore, the workshop will also consider other potential synergistic actions of vitamins.

The prevailing opinion is that a so-called balanced diet provides all essential nutrients in adequate amounts (RDAs). However, the intake necessary to cover additional functions adequately may not be achieved with such a balanced diet unless special measures are taken to adapt the dietary behaviour specifically. Guidelines advising a much higher intake of fruits and vegetables (5–7 servings per day) have already been established to help in the reduction of risk for certain diseases such as some types of cancer, coronary heart disease and maybe also the degeneration of mental functions (e.g. Parkinson and Alzheimer disease). Such a diet includes several vitamins at considerably higher amounts than the respective RDAs, e.g. about 200 mg vitamin C, 20–30 IU vitamin E, 6 mg β-carotene and also several of the B vitamins such as folate and vitamin B_6. It is quite likely that these increased intakes of vitamins together with other nutrients may play an important role for the beneficial effect of such a diet rich in fruit and vegetables.

But even when these special guidelines are followed it may not be possible to adequately cover particular additional needs for some of the vitamins. The most typical example is the prevention of neural tube defect by folate. Thus it may be necessary to take special measures to adequately cover these additional needs.

Today, individuals are very much concerned about their personal contribution to well-being and 'optimal' health in later life. Guidelines advising what to eat according to the latest established scientific information on vitamins and other nutrients to reduce the risk for certain diseases are in demand by a broad segment of the population. Since knowledge accumulates rapidly, such guidelines should be reassessed frequently to incorporate new scientific data, and competent organizations such as academies or other professional associations could be responsible to establish them. These could now and even more so in the future contribute to lower public health costs by contributing to the reduction of the incidence of costly chronic diseases.

Since many of the leading experts attended the workshop it was decided to publish not only the lectures but also summaries of the discussions in the working groups. For the topics of each session, one working group was formed. They were asked to include in their discussions and summaries the following four questions: (1) Do we have sufficient evidence to make recommendations for increasing the current allowance of vitamins to beneficially effect certain functions? (2) What knowledge is missing before new vitamin recommendations for optimal function can be developed? (3) How long will it take to obtain the missing knowledge? (4) How should our current knowledge be communicated to the consumer?

Finally it should be mentioned that like the previous workshop on 'The Scientific Basis for Vitamin Intake in Human Nutrition' [1], this meeting was also organized in the name of the European Academy of Nutritional Sciences and was held in October 1997. The contents of this book represent a continuation of the discussions held in the previous volume.

Reference

1 Walter P (ed): The Scientific Basis for Vitamin Intake in Human Nutrition. Bibl Nutr Dieta. Basel, Karger, 1995, vol 52.

Prof. Paul Walter, Swiss Vitamin Institute and Department of Biochemistry,
University of Basel, Vesalgasse 1, CH–4051 Basel (Switzerland)
E-Mail paul.walter@unibas.ch

Walter P, Hornig D, Moser U (eds): Functions of Vitamins beyond Recommended Dietary Allowances. Bibl Nutr Dieta. Basel, Karger, 2001, No 55, pp 4–13

Dietary Reference Intakes: A New Approach to Setting Nutrition Standards in the USA and Canada

Allison A. Yates

Food and Nutrition Board, Institute of Medicine, National Academy of Sciences, Washington, D.C., USA

It is a great pleasure to be here to discuss the progress to date on the Dietary Reference Intake initiative. This presentation covers three areas: (1) the present status of vitamin recommendations in the United States and Canada, (2) what the ideas are for setting upper safe levels, and (3) the time scale for everything that is planned.

Development of the Framework

Since 1992, the Food and Nutrition Board (FNB) in the United States has been undergoing an extensive review of (1) the process for developing nutrient-based dietary recommendations and reference intakes and (2) the uses made of quantitative estimates of intakes. When the previous meeting of the EANS was held in 1994 [1], the FNB had just issued a comment paper entitled 'How Should the Recommended Dietary Allowances be Revised?' [2]. It put forward a framework for developing dietary allowances and other quantitative reference intakes patterned to a large extent on the previous Dietary Reference Values of the United Kingdom [3], in which four reference values were given: a lower intake at which a high probability of deficiency existed, an estimated average requirement, a recommended intake, and an upper safe level of intake.

The definition of an RDA has remained somewhat the same for many years [4], and has not changed in the new framework as described here. The ideal criteria for establishing a recommended intake is to select a healthy, representative sample of the population, determine the average requirements of that group; assess the range of individual variability, and calculate an allowance to cover needs. The new term, Dietary Reference Intakes (or DRIs), is a collective term that includes four nutrient-based dietary reference values. The values are the Estimated Average Requirement (EAR), Recommended Dietary Allowance (RDA), Adequate Intake (AI), and Tolerable Upper Intake Level (UL). As is evident, some of these are similar, but in total these do not parallel the Dietary Reference Values of the United Kingdom [3]. In addition, a key concept included in the comment paper [2] was that the recommended intakes would not necessarily be restricted to being developed based on criteria related to prevention of nutrient deficiency diseases, but also to levels of intake which were expected to decrease risk of chronic disease *where the data were conclusive.*

Based on comments received to that initial proposal, adjustments were made in the proposed framework, as described in this discussion; but of significance is the continued inclusion of basing recommended intakes on risk of all diseases or chronic conditions, rather than focusing only on deficiency diseases.

Also of importance in the development of this new framework was the subsequent recognition by the FNB, based on an earlier report of the FNB on using recommended intakes to assess nutrient adequacy [5], that RDAs would not refer to population goals, but would be more accurately goals for individuals. This is in keeping with both the growing understanding of the influence of the variability of intakes in evaluating population intakes, and a better understanding that in estimating average requirements, it is an estimate for an individual. Given the concerns as discussed in the 1994 EANS Workshop [1] with regard to the growing body of evidence indicating the role of nutrients and other substances in food on long-term health, mounting interest developed on the part of federal agencies in the United States and Canada to provide funding to undertake the development of new dietary allowances which would apply the new framework to one group of nutrients, as a trial/test of the model (fig. 1).

With the involvement of the Health Protection Branch of Health Canada, the US Department of Health and Human Services agencies (Office of Undersecretary for Health, the Food and Drug Administration, and the National Heart, Lung and Blood Institute at NIH), and the US Department of Agriculture contracted with the FNB to initiate the project. In December 1995, the National Academy of Sciences appointed a standing committee to oversee this process. The Standing Committee on the Scientific Evaluation of Dietary Reference Intakes currently has ten members, one of whom is from Canada. It is hoped that the government of Mexico can also participate in future portions of the process.

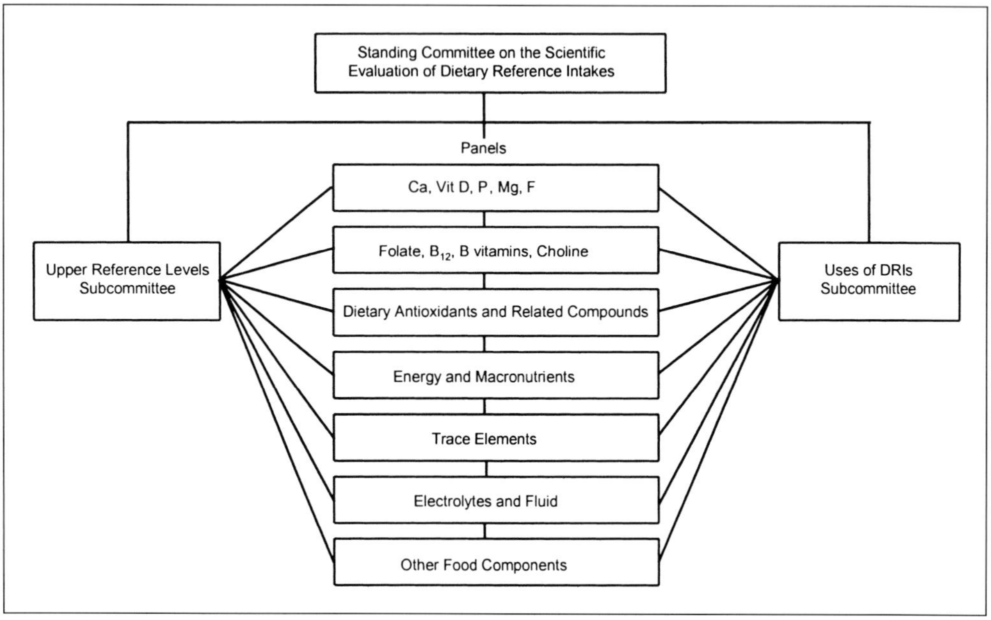

Fig. 1. Dietary Reference Intakes.

Initiation of the DRI Process

The first panel, the Panel on Calcium and Related Nutrients, was formed in early 1996. Their charge was to evaluate the scientific literature and establish, where adequate data was available, estimated average requirements for subgroups varying in age and gender, determine the variability of such requirements, and then develop recommended dietary allowances of levels of intake which would be the minimal amounts necessary to maintain approximately 98% of individuals in a population subgroup at the criterion of adequacy. The first group of nutrients so evaluated included calcium, phosphorus, magnesium, vitamin D, and fluoride [6].

Simultaneously with this effort, the Subcommittee on Upper Reference Levels was appointed. Their charge was to develop a model of risk assessment for nutrients, using standard risk assessment methodology, but adapted to the fact that nutrients are required for normal metabolism and thus are not contaminants, for which it is expected that one would want to have as low a level in the diet as possible. They were to apply the model to develop upper levels of intake of the five nutrients included in this first group that, when consumed chronically, would not result in adverse effects in more sensitive members of the population subgroup.

What are the Dietary Reference Intakes?

The overall framework has been titled *Dietary Reference Intakes.* DRIs are a set of reference values that can be used for planning and assessing diets for healthy populations and for many other purposes. They expand upon and replace the RDAs, which have been published since 1941 by the National Academy of Sciences [4], and are intended to replace the Recommended Nutrient Intakes developed in Canada [7]. As mentioned earlier, DRIs encompass the EAR, RDA, AI and UL.

Estimated Average Requirement

The EAR is the nutrient value that is estimated to meet the requirement defined by a specified indicator of adequacy in 50% of the individuals in a life stage and gender group. At this level of intake, the remaining 50% of the specified group would not have their nutrient needs met. For some life stage or gender groups, data may have to be extrapolated to estimate this value. In deriving the EARs, contemporary concepts of the reduction of disease risk are among the factors considered, rather than basing reference values solely upon the prevention of nutrient deficiencies. The EAR is used in setting the RDA, and it may be used as one factor for assessing the adequacy of intakes of groups and for planning adequate intakes by groups.

Recommended Dietary Allowance

The RDA is the daily dietary intake level that is sufficient to meet the nutrient requirements of nearly all (97–98%) individuals in the life stage and gender group. The RDA applies to individuals, not to groups. The EAR serves as the foundation for setting the RDA. If the standard deviation (SD) of the EAR is available, the RDA is set at 2 SDs above the EAR:

$$RDA = EAR + 2\ SD_{EAR}.$$

If data about variability in requirements are insufficient to calculate a standard deviation, a coefficient of variation (CV_{EAR}) of 10% is assumed, and the resulting equation for the RDA is:

$$RDA = EAR + 2(EAR \times 0.1)$$
$$RDA = EAR \times (1.2).$$

If data are sufficient only to set an AI (see discussion following) for a nutrient for a specific life stage group, no RDA will be set.

Adequate Intake

If sufficient scientific evidence is not available to calculate an EAR, a value called an AI is used instead. The AI is based on observed or experimentally determined approximations of a nutrient intake, by a defined population or subgroup, that appear to sustain a defined nutritional state, such as normal circulating nutrient values or growth. In the case of young infants, for whom human milk is the recommended sole source of food for the first 4–6 months of life, the AI is based on the daily nutrient intake supplied by human milk for healthy, full-term infants who are exclusively breast-fed.

The AI may be expected to exceed the EAR and possibly the RDA for the same specified endpoints of nutritional adequacy. The AI value depends upon the indicator of nutritional adequacy, the dietary characteristics of the group used to derive it, and the database and methods used to estimate it. Therefore, the excess of an AI, relative to a true EAR, is likely to differ among nutrients, population groups, and distinct sociocultural settings. In the absence of definitive data on which to base an EAR and RDA, the AI may be used as a goal for nutrient intake of individuals.

It should be emphasized that the AI as defined above is different from both the RDA and from the WHO 'lower limit of the population mean intake range for nutritional sufficiency', which are each based on a determined EAR [8].

In the first report issued on calcium, phosphorus, magnesium, vitamin D and fluoride, AIs rather than EARs and RDAs have been proposed for all nutrients for infants to the age of 1 year, and for calcium, vitamin D, and fluoride for all other life stages.

Vitamin D, an Example of a Case Where an AI is the Recommended Intake (table 1). For vitamin D, as an example, the AI is the intake value that appears to be needed to maintain, in a defined group of individuals with limited and uncertain sun exposure and stores, circulating serum 25-OH-vitamin D concentrations above a defined amount [6]. Here the rationale for an AI rather than EAR was that methods are not available to determine the extent to which stores are being used, or that sun exposure is providing additional sources. The cutoff for serum 25-OH-vitamin D was the concentration below which vitamin D deficiency rickets or osteomalacia occurs in some individuals. The intake value was rounded to the nearest 50 IU in micrograms, and then doubled as a safety factor to cover the needs of all, regardless of exposure to the sun.

Indicator of Nutrient Adequacy

Since the publication of the last version of the Recommended Dietary Allowances in the United States [4], the Canadian Recommended Nutrient Intakes [7], and the report on *Diet and Health* [9], the research base related to the role of diet in chronic disease has expanded sufficiently to permit moving beyond deficiency indicators to other indicators with broader functional significance. Examples of such indicators are those related to decreasing the

Table 1. Criteria and AI values for vitamin D by life stage group

	Criterion	AI, μg/day[a–c]
Life stage group		
0–6 months	Human milk	5
7–12 months	Human milk	5
1 through 50 years	Serum 25(OH)D	5
51 through 70 years	Serum 25(OH)D	10
>70 years	Serum 25(OH)D	15
Pregnancy		
<18 years	Serum 25(OH)D	5
19 through 50 years	Serum 25(OH)D	5
Lactation		
<18 years	Serum 25(OH)D	5
19 through 50 years	Serum 25(OH)D	5

[a] All groups except Pregnancy and Lactation are males and females.
[b] As cholecalciferol. 1 μg cholecalciferol = 40 IU vitamin D.
[c] In the absence of adequate exposure to sunlight.

risk of chronic diseases such as osteoporosis, heart disease, or hypertension. However, there is insufficient scientific evidence to relate every nutrient to functional indicators of chronic disease, and it cannot be expected that all nutrients will be related to a chronic disease, condition, or developmental abnormality. In using such indicators, it becomes critical to establish concordance of data of various types. Thus what is observed in the laboratory experimentally should also be observed in appropriately conducted clinical trials and observational studies of populations.

Criteria for Dietary Reference Intakes

Until more is known about the prevalence of chronic disease risk and habitual nutrient intakes in other countries, the implications of these DRIs should be used with caution outside the United States and Canada. Associations may not be easily identified in short-term studies where requirements are based on estimated intakes to decrease risk of disease, particularly chronic disease.

It is important to recognize that the major focus in the development of EARs and AIs has been the determination of the most appropriate indicator of adequacy. Once this is determined, then, from data available, the EAR or AI is derived. A key question is 'adequate for what?'. The value derived for the EAR, for example, would differ depending on the functional outcome that was judged to be the most relevant based on the scientific data available. Each EAR and AI is described in terms of the functional endpoint or outcome that it is developed to address.

Criteria and Proposed Values for Tolerable Upper Intake Levels

The UL is the maximal level of nutrient intake that is unlikely to pose risks of adverse health effects to almost all individuals in the target group. The term 'tolerable intake' was chosen to avoid implying a possible beneficial effect. Instead, the term is intended to connote a level of intake that can, with high probability, be tolerated biologically. The UL is not intended to be a recommended level of intake, and there is no established benefit for healthy individuals associated with nutrient intakes above the RDA or AI.

The need to set ULs grew out of the increase in the practice of fortifying foods with nutrients and in the use of dietary supplements by more people and in larger doses. For most nutrients, the UL refers to total intakes from food, fortified food, and nutrient supplements. In some instances, it may refer only to intakes from pharmacological preparations. The UL applies to chronic daily use.

The model developed is a risk assessment model that consists of a systematic series of scientific considerations and judgments to be used in deriving a UL. The hallmark of the risk assessment model is the requirement to be explicit in all the evaluations and judgments that must be made to document conclusions. Primarily due to limitations of the database, ULs are set for very broad age groups.

The model requires the determination of a Lowest Observed Adverse Effect Level (LOAEL) of intake, and some understanding of a No Observed Adverse Effect Level (NOAEL). An uncertainty factor (UF) is developed that is based on a review of the data available regarding the nutrient and its relationship to the LOAEL and NOAEL. Depending on the severity of the adverse effect noted, the number of individuals in whom adverse effects have been described, the source and environment of the nutrient, and other factors in the diet that affect the nutrient, the UF may be somewhat large or very small.

In the case of vitamin D, in order to develop a UL, data were available to establish a LOAEL for adults based on the adverse effect of hypercalcemia (defined as a serum calcium level >2.75 mmol/l (11 mg/dl)) at 95 μg (3,800 IU) per day. The NOAEL determined was 60 μg (2,400 IU) as observed in adults. Given the uncertainties in the data reviewed, a UF of 1.2 was chosen for adults. This resulted in a UL of 60 μg/1.2 ≈ 50 μg (2,000 IU)/day.

The UL values have been set to protect the most sensitive individuals in the healthy general population (such as elderly individuals who tend to have a decreased glomerular filtration rate). They are likely to be too high for persons with certain illnesses (such as, in the case of vitamin D, renal glomerular disease) or genetic abnormalities that affect the utilization or decrease the elimination of the nutrient.

Next Nutrient Groups to Be Reviewed

Currently, the panel on folate, B vitamins, and choline is developing their report, which is expected to be completed by April 1998. The panel is not only looking at levels needed to decrease risk of deficiencies, but also at levels necessary to effect development of chronic disease and developmental abnormalities.

Here new concerns arise with respect to the vitamins under study: as brought out in workshops held by the panel, to what extent should DRIs be developed for an entire population subgroup when subgroups within that segment of the population have genotypically determined requirements that are not shared by most of the population? To what extent can DRIs be developed which include all who appear to be healthy? Also, as one looks at aging, what is 'normal' for a 75-year-old? Is lack of intrinsic factor due to achlorhydria normal, or a clinical pathology? Data are needed on prevalence to decide how to approach the development of average requirements in such situations.

Timeline

Given the level of complexity for this process, it is understandable that all nutrients and food components cannot be reviewed simultaneously. We have recently begun the third group of nutrients, dietary antioxidants and related compounds; this panel, which has not been appointed yet, will have as its first charge to define the criteria to be used to determine which nutrients and food components should be included in this review of dietary antioxidants, and develop a list of compounds to review, knowing that it will review at a minimum β-carotene, vitamin C, and vitamin E (these were required in the contractual agreement with the funding agencies). It is expected that additional substances will be reviewed, in all probability selenium and other carotenoids, but that will not be decided until after the panel has deliberated, held a workshop on the topic, and developed an initial report. The final report on

Dietary Antioxidants was due in September 1999. Polyunsaturated fatty acids will be included in this report to the extent of providing one aspect of determining oxidative stress.

The other functional groups of nutrients and food components are in various stages of development. It is expected that energy and macronutrients will be next, but this is all based on funding availability. The overall process is expected to cost about USD 6 million, and to date about USD 2.7 million has been received. It is hoped that with timely funding, the remaining four groups can be reviewed by the end of the year 2000. Then it will be possible to go back and periodically review or update specific nutrients or food components when new data accumulates without having to review the entire group. With today's publishing techniques, there is little reason not to have periodic updates that are more timely than every 5–10 years.

Of critical importance to the usability of the DRI framework is the work of the Subcommittee on Uses of Dietary Reference Intakes; although it is important to develop the scientific basis for using the quantitative estimates derived, it is equally important to evaluate their appropriate uses in the two major roles for dietary recommendations: setting goals for individuals and populations, and assessing adequacy of intake for individuals and populations.

The report on calcium and related nutrients [6] and the process described have focused on the database used to justify the estimates of reference intakes, which is the intended use of the report as currently funded. However, although many scientists and policymakers pay specific attention to the database needed to develop the recommended and reference intakes, many more health professionals use them in various ways to serve as the basis for counseling, nutrition education, etc. It is thus just as important for the FNB to undertake additional initiatives to provide significant guidance regarding the use of the various reference values and the categories of DRIs, as it is to emphasize the need to review the data in depth in order to develop them.

References

1 Walter P (ed): The scientific basis for vitamin intake in human nutrition. Bibl Nutr Dieta. Basel, Karger, 1995, vol 52.

2 Institute of Medicine: How Should the Recommended Dietary Intakes Be Revised? Food and Nutrition Board. Washington, National Academy Press, 1994.

3 Committee on Medical Aspects of Food Policy: Dietary Reference Values for Food Energy and Nutrients for the United Kingdom. Report on Health and Social Subjects, No 41. London, HMSO, 1991.

4 National Research Council: Recommended Dietary Allowances, ed 10. Report of the Subcommittee on the Tenth Edition of the RDAs, Food and Nutrition Board, Commission on Life Sciences. Washington, National Academy Press, 1989.

5 National Research Council: Nutrient Adequacy: Assessment Using Food Consumption Surveys. Washington, National Academy Press, 1986.
6 Institute of Medicine: Dietary Reference Intakes for Calcium, Phosphorus, Magnesium, Vitamin D, and Fluoride. Standing Committee on the Scientific Evaluation of Dietary Reference Intakes, Food and Nutrition Board, Institute of Medicine. Washington, National Academy Press, 1997.
7 Health and Welfare Canada: Nutrition Recommendations. The Report of the Scientific Review Committee 1990. Ottawa, Canadian Government Publishing Centre, 1990.
8 World Health Organization: Trace Elements in Human Nutrition and Health. Prepared in collaboration with the Food and Agriculture Organization of the United Nations and the International Atomic Energy Agency. Geneva, WHO, 1996.
9 National Research Council: Diet and Health: Implications for Reducing Chronic Disease Risk. Report of the Committee on Diet and Health, Food and Nutrition Board, Commission on Life Sciences. Washington, National Academy Press, 1989.

Dr. Allison A. Yates, Institute of Medicine, National Academy of Sciences,
2101 Constitution Ave, NW, Washington, DC 20418 (USA)
Tel. +1 202 334 1732, Fax +1 202 334 2316, E-Mail ayates@nas.edu

Walter P, Hornig D, Moser U (eds): Functions of Vitamins beyond Recommended Dietary Allowances. Bibl Nutr Dieta. Basel, Karger, 2001, No 55, pp 14–21

Recommendations for Vitamin Intake in the European Union and the Use of Reference Values in Existing and Future Community Legislation

Basil Mathioudakis

European Commission, Directorate-General on Industry, Unit III.E.1 – Foodstuffs – Legislation: Scientific and Technical Aspects, Brussels, Belgium

Almost all Member States of the European Union and many other European countries have recommendations for the intake of nutrients and more specifically for the intake of vitamins. These recommendations have been derived by Committees of experts convened independently by the responsible national instances.

In reaching their recommendations, some of these Committees examined mainly original scientific data, others reviewed recommendations of other Committees and yet others did both [1]. At the end of the 1980s and as the programme of food harmonization in view of the establishment of the Internal Market in the European Community was advancing, the need was felt for such recommendations at Community level. It was felt also that there was no reason to assume that basic nutrient requirements were different across the Community. This was supported by the fact that for most nutrients the recommendations from different national committees were fairly similar.

The European Commission asked therefore the Scientific Committee for Food (SCF) to advise on the establishment of Recommended Dietary Allowances for Nutrients in the European Community and to make recommendations.

A high number of ad-hoc experts were invited to assist the SCF in its task. These experts had either considerable overall experience in the development of recommendations in different Member States or expertise in individual nutrients and together with the members of the SCF constituted an excellent

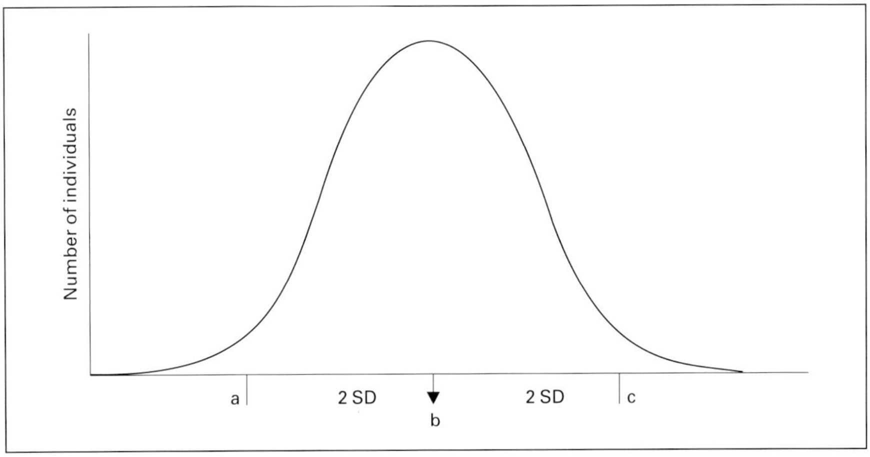

Fig. 1. The frequency distribution of individual requirements for a nutrient.

representative body in the field across the Community. Their opinion was expressed on December 1992 [2].

The SCF considered the reports and drew on the experience of expert Committees of Member States, of third countries and of international organizations. However, their report did not constitute a summary or a combination or a compromise of other reports but was the result of consideration of the most up-to-date data and on decisions based on the interpretation of these data.

The Committee accepted to make the basic assumption that nutrient requirements of individuals have a gaussian distribution with the average requirement as the peak, although not much experimental evidence in support of this assumption was available (fig. 1). It chose however to get away from the practice of recommending a single value because such single values were often misinterpreted or misused. It attempted to give, where possible, three values which correspond to points c, b and a in figure 1. These are defined as follows:

Lowest Threshold Intake (LTI) is the intake below which, on the basis of current knowledge, almost all individuals will be unlikely to maintain metabolic integrity according to the criterion chosen for each nutrient. This value corresponds to point a.

Average Requirement (AR) for a group corresponds to point b.

Population Reference Intake (PRI) is the intake which will meet the needs of virtually all healthy people in a group corresponding to point c. This value corresponds conceptually to the values which bear names such as recom-

Table 1. Multiple values for vitamins proposed for adults in the European Community (amounts per day, unless given in other terms; if that for women is different from that for men, it is given in parentheses)

Nutrient	Average requirement	Population reference intake	Lowest threshold intake
Vitamin A, µg	500 (400)	700 (600)	300 (250)
Thiamin, mg	0.8 (0.6) 72 µg/MJ	1.1 (0.9) 100 µg/MJ	 50 µg/MJ
Riboflavin, mg	1.3 (1.1)	1.6 (1.3)	0.6
Niacin, mg niacin equivalents	15 (11) 1.3/MJ	18 (14) 1.6/MJ	 1.0/MJ
Vitamin B_6, mg	1.3 (1.0) 13 µg/g protein	1.5 (1.1) 15 µg/g protein	–
Folate, µg	140	200[1]	85
Vitamin B_{12}, µg	1.0	1.4	0.6
Vitamin C, mg	30	45	12
Vitamin E, mg α-tocopherol equivalents		0.4 µg/g PUFA	4 (3)/day regardless of PUFA intakes

PUFA = Polyunsaturated fatty acids.

[1] Neural tube effects have been shown to be prevented in offspring by periconceptual ingestion of 400 µg folic acid per day in the form of supplements.

For the following, acceptable ranges of intake are given:

Pantothenic acid, mg	3–12
Biotin, µg	15–100
Vitamin D, µg	0–10

mended daily amounts, recommended daily allowances, recommended daily intakes, recommended dietary intakes, recommended nutrient intakes etc. adopted by other committees.

The PRI is usually considered as the mean +2 standard deviation which would cover the needs of 97.5% of the population in the group. The SCF said that the given value incorporates safety factors and therefore adequately covers the needs of all individuals in the group. For those vitamins for which a PRI could not be established, a range of safe and adequate intakes was given. The proposals for vitamins are summarized in table 1.

The process of assessing the requirements for a nutrient depends on the choice of the determinant parameter of adequacy. It also depends on the choice of the levels for adequacy. The choice of the parameters and of the adequacy levels which in effect are arbitrary influence the final result.

Further, in determining the PRI or otherwise named but conceptually corresponding values, political, economical, social and national or regional health factors may be taken into account. These may differ from one Member State of the Community to the other and can explain the small differences between the values derived by the SCF for the European Community and those derived by national authorities for specific populations. For example, in the very recent report on the Recommended Dietary Allowances for Ireland, an RDA for iron for children which is higher than the corresponding PRI for the European Community is recommended because of high incidence of iron deficiency anaemia in children and young adolescent females in Ireland [3]. The same reason influences recommending a higher value for vitamin C which increases non-haem iron absorption. Differences for the above reasons should be clearly distinguished from those due to availability of new scientific evidence which is the reason given in the Irish report as justification for a higher value for calcium.

The PRIs have generally been based upon the principle of prevention of deficiencies and this is valid for the values adopted by the SCF and for those adopted by national committees. Work on the relationships between nutrient intake and reduction of risk to disease have not been taken into account although such work has been acknowledged. In the German recommendations for example it is stated that 'At present, special attention is devoted to the antioxidative effects of vitamins C and E and of carotenoids in the control of diseases. However, the present state of knowledge does not yet justify more specific recommendations' [4]. The UK report states that 'claims have also been made that at very high levels of intake some nutrients have especially beneficial or therapeutic effects but the Panel decided that these effects did not fall within their definition of requirement' [5]. The SCF in its report marks the PRI of 200 μg for folic acid with the statement that 'neural tube defects have been shown to be prevented in offspring by periconceptual ingestion of 400 μg folic acid per day in the form of supplements', admits that it is difficult to justify a requirement for vitamin C in excess of tissue storage capacity and express the hope 'that in the future more information will become available on the quantitative role of vitamin C in the body's defences against free radicals and on epidemiological evidence that appears to link higher vitamin C intakes with a lower incidence of some disease' and notes that 'claims that very generous intakes of vitamin E have beneficial effects on health are not taken into account in making the present recommendations'. Maybe the Irish Nutrition Committee is making a first small step when trying to explain an Irish

RDA for vitamin C which is higher than the PRI for the European Community, it uses as one of the arguments the fact that 'there is evidence to suggest that higher vitamin C intakes may lower the risk of some chronic diseases such as cataract, cancer and cardiovascular diseases'.

The Commission asked the SCF to advise on the establishment of values which would be used for a number of purposes. The SCF bore that in mind and felt that multiple values were of greater utility than just a simple one. Such values can be used for prescribing diets or provisions of food supplies, for assessing the diet of groups, for assessing the diet of individuals and for other scientific purposes which have been discussed by experts in the field. This paper will concentrate on the use of such values in existing and possible future Community legislation.

Since 1985 the new approach on food legislation is a horizontal approach, that is stipulating provisions which are applicable across the whole range of foodstuffs. Few are the areas where specific directives (vertical directives) are in force or envisaged. The essential criteria for selecting these areas are 'the protection of health and life of humans' referred to in Article 36 of the Treaty of Rome and 'essential requirements' which could also justifiably override the application of the principle of free movement of goods enshrined in Article 30 of the same Treaty. Further it has been specified that provisions likely to have an effect on public health shall be adopted after consultation of the SCF. In this context the Commission has adopted or is planning to adopt in the future a number of specific directives in the area of foods for particular nutritional uses comprising essential compositional requirement which are or will be based on relevant reports of the SCF.

The essential composition of infant formulae and follow-on formulae was based, in accordance with the opinion of the SCF [6], on the average composition of human milk which is used, taking into account its consumption by wholly breast-fed infants, for determining the requirement of artificially fed infants.

For weaning foods, no great consideration has been given to fixing minimum requirements for vitamins. With very few exceptions it was considered that the natural composition of this category of varied products was sufficient. However, when the SCF was requested to advise on the maximum levels for vitamins in these products it used the PRIs established for young children and recommended that certain intake levels related to these PRIs should not be exceeded per specified amount of the weaning food [7]. These recommendations have been taken up by the Commission services and are included in the draft legislation on the subject currently under discussion with the Member States.

Food intended for use in energy-restricted diets for weight reduction are covered by Commission Directive 96/8/EC [8]. Such products can be used as replacement for the whole of the daily diet or as replacement for one or more meals of the daily diet. Annex I of the directive lays down the essential composition of these products. Paragraph 5 of Annex I stipulates that products used as replacement of the whole of the daily diet should contain at least 100% of amounts of vitamins which are specified in a table while products used as replacement of a meal should contain 30% of these amounts. In its opinion which was adopted in October 1990, the SCF recommended that these reference amounts should be the PRIs which at the time were being developed by the same Committee [9] and indeed these were the values included in the directive when adopted in February 1996.

Another specific directive foreseen for adoption by Annex I of Directive 89/398/EEC concerns foods for special medical purposes (FSMP). In view of preparing the relevant draft the European Commission requested the opinion of the SCF on, among others, the essential compositional requirements of FSMPs. In its opinion [10] the SCF recommended that these products in general should provide such amounts of vitamins that for an assumed energy intake of 2,000 kcal from these products they would also ensure at least the EU PRI for adult males (>18 years). Of course, given the particular nature of these products, a series of exceptions are stipulated as necessary in the SCF's opinion. It is interesting to note that the SCF recommends that in the absence of EU PRIs the US RDAs be used as reference values and in the absence of those that the acceptable ranges of intake should be used as corresponding minima and maxima. The SCF also felt that for these products it would be wise to fix upper limits too and as a general rule suggested this limit to be 300% of the EU PRI or the US RDA as the case may be. The Commission services in preparing the relevant draft-specific directive will, as always, consider with great attention the recommendations of the SCF.

Nutrition labelling in the European Union is governed by directive 90/496/EEC [11] adopted in 1990. Article 6, paragraph 2 and 5a specify that information on vitamins be expressed per 100 g or per 100 ml and as a percentage of the reference values given in the Annex of that directive. These reference values are the same included in the Codex Guidelines on Nutrition Labelling [12]. These values were established by a Joint FAO/WHO Consultation specially convened [13] and although they were called 'Nutrient Reference Values' they in fact represented the RDAs. They were used in the absence of any specific Community recommendations on this issue at the time.

In its report on nutrient and energy intakes for the European Community, the SCF specifically considered the choice of the reference value for nutrition labelling in itself and whether different values should be recommended for different groups of the population.

The SCF recognized that such choices involved more than strictly scientific considerations. It was also aware that, traditionally, reference values for nutrition labelling correspond with the PRI for adult male proposed value. It considered the arguments in favour of this approach and those in favour of the view that such value would be too high as a nutrition labelling reference value. It finally recommended to use as reference value the Average Requirement for adult men which would cover the need of the majority of the population with two exceptions. For iron it proposed in addition a higher reference value for women (14 mg) than the one for men (7 mg) and for vitamin D, in the absence of an AR value, it proposed the midpoint of the acceptable intake for adults, namely 5 μg. The recommendations of the SCF have not yet found their way into Community legislation but this is due to administrative reasons and do not reflect at this stage any judgement on the recommendations by the European Commission and the Member States. Due consideration is expected to be given to them in forthcoming discussions in the context of a wider revision of the Community nutrition labelling rules.

The SCF felt that a separate set of nutrition labelling values was necessary for the labelling of products intended specifically for the particular nutritional use by infants and young children. They based those values on the PRIs for infants and young children between 6 months and 3 years. This recommendation was incorporated recently into Community legislation concerning relevant products [14, 15].

Legislation on food supplements and on the addition of nutrients to foods is at present not harmonized at Community level. The national rules are very diverse but the concept of RDAs is central to the majority of these rules. In some Member States it is compulsory to add vitamins A and D to margarine. The minimum level per 100 g of the product are very near to the RDA values for the adult population for vitamin A (Denmark 840 μg/100 g, Ireland 900 μg/100 g, UK 800 μg/100 g, Sweden 900 μg/100 g). The minimum levels imposed for vitamin D (Ireland 7.5 μg/100 g, UK 7.5 μg/100 g, Sweden 7.5 μg/100 g) are very near the recommended levels for some vulnerable groups of the population although as a whole a range is usually proposed for vitamin D. This range for the Community lies between 0 and 10 μg.

For noncompulsory additions, those national legislations which impose limits to the addition of nutrients set those limits as multiples of the applicable RDA or PRI. This is the case for example in Belgium and Greece. The same approach is also adopted for setting minimum and maximum levels for vitamin content in food supplements.

The Commission circulated in June 1997 a discussion paper in view of a possible harmonization of legislation in these two subjects [16]. The paper raises the most important points that need to be considered and debated prior to any proposals for harmonization. One of those is certainly the subject of upper limits for nutrients added to foods or contained in food supplements and whether such limits should be based on safety or on nutritional considerations as represented by the PRI.

It has been demonstrated above that the various reference values which have been proposed for the European Community have been or will be very useful for establishing certain Community legal rules. However, as stated earlier, these values may be used for a variety of other purposes, some of which may require the incorporation of some nonscientific factors in the determination of these values. This may explain why some national reference values may continue to differ somewhat from those recommended for the Community.

References

1 Trichopoulou A, Vassilakou T: Recommended dietary intakes in the European Community Member States: An overview. Eur J Clin Nutr 1990 (suppl 2):51–126.

2 Reports of the Scientific Community for Food, 31st Series: Nutrient and Energy Intakes for the European Community. Luxembourg, Office for Official Publications of the European Communities, 1993.

3 Report to the Minister for Health: Recommended Dietary Allowances for Ireland. Dublin, Nutrition Committee of the Food Safety Advisory Board, 1997.

4 Recommendations on Nutrient Intake, Abstracts and Tables, ed 5. Frankfurt, German Society of Nutrition, 1991.

5 Report on Health and Social Subjects No 41: Dietary Reference Values for Food Energy and Nutrients for the UK. London, HMSO, 1991.

6 Reports of the Scientific Committee for Food, 14th Series: First report on the essential requirements of infant formulae and follow-up milks based on cow's milk proteins. Luxembourg, Office for Official Publications of the European Communities, 1983.

7 Report of the Scientific Committee for Food: Maximum limits for vitamins and minerals in processed cereal-based food and baby foods (to be published).

8 Commission Directive 96/8/EC on foods intended for use in energy-restricted diets for weight reduction. Official Journal of the European Communities No L 55 of 06.03.1996, pp 22–26.

9 Reports of the Scientific Committee for Food, 27th Series: Foods intended for weight control diets. Luxembourg, Office for Official Publications of the European Communities, 1992.

10 Reports of the Scientific Committee for Food: Foods for special medical purposes (to be published).

11 Council Directive 90/496/EEC on nutrition labelling for foodstuffs. Official Journal of the European Communities. No L 276 of 06.10.1990, pp 40–44.

12 Codex Alimentarius: Vol 1 – Suppl 1: Guidelines on Nutrition Labelling. Rome, Food and Agriculture Organisation of the United Nations, 1993.

13 Report of a joint FAO/WHO expert consultation on recommended allowances of nutrients for food labelling purposes. Rome, Food and Agriculture Organisation of the United Nations, 1988.

14 Commission Directive 96/4/EC amending Directive 91/321/EEC on infant formulae and follow-on formulae. Official Journal of The European Communities No L 49 of 28.02.1996, pp 12–16.

15 Commission Directive 96/5/EEC on processed cereal-based foods and baby foods for infants and young children. Official Journal of the European Communities No L 49 of 28.02.1996, pp 17–28.

16 Discussion Paper III/5934/97 on addition of vitamins and minerals to foods and on food supplements. Brussels, European Commission, 1997.

Dr. Basil Mathioudakis, Directorate-General Industry, Commission of the European Communities, Rue de la Loi, 200, B–1049 Brussels (Belgium)
Tel. +32 2 295 9182, Fax +32 2 295 1735

Walter P, Hornig D, Moser U (eds): Functions of Vitamins beyond Recommended Dietary Allowances. Bibl Nutr Dieta. Basel, Karger, 2001, No 55, pp 22–33

Folic Acid and Neural Tube Defects

Nicholas J. Wald

Department of Environmental and Preventive Medicine, Wolfson Institute of Preventive Medicine, St Bartholomew's and the Royal London School of Medicine and Dentistry, London, UK

The Importance of Fortifying Food with Folic Acid

At the meeting of the European Academy of Nutritional Sciences in Cannes in 1995, the evidence on folic acid and neural tube defects was reviewed and the reasons were given why the main method of prevention should be the fortification of a staple food, such as flour, with folic acid [Wald, 1995]. In brief, there was conclusive evidence from randomised controlled trials with supporting data from observational studies and nonrandomised trials that neural tube defects are a folate deficiency disorder. Taking extra folic acid had been shown to prevent about three-quarters of neural tube defects. It had also been recognised by public health authorities that intakes of folic acid needed to be increased. Three approaches could be adopted to increase folic acid consumption: (1) women planning a pregnancy could take folic acid supplements; (2) women could eat folate-rich foods, such as green leafy vegetables, and orange juice, and (3) a staple food, such as bread or flour, could be fortified with folic acid.

About half of all pregnancies are unplanned, so that even if all women planning a pregnancy took a folic acid supplement, a large proportion of women would remain unprotected. The necessary change in folate intake required to achieve significant reduction in the birth prevalence of neural tube defects (about 0.4 mg folic acid daily) would require a substantial dietary change that would be impractical without a food-fortifying policy. This assessment was confirmed by Cuskelly et al. [1966] who compared the efficiency of using folate-rich foods with supplements and fortified food as means of increasing folate status. Their results, displayed in figure 1, showed that advice to

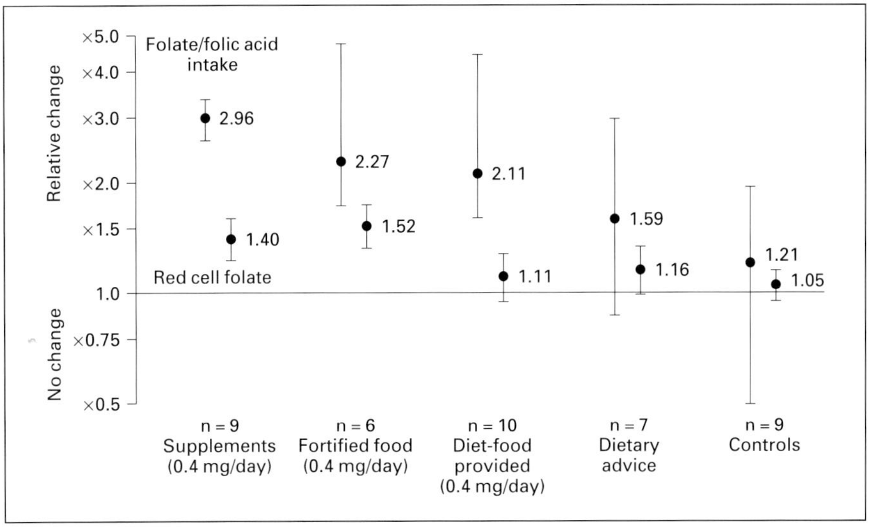

Fig. 1. Effect of changes in dietary folate/folic acid on red cell folate adapted from Cuskelly et al. [1996].

women to consume folate-rich foods as a means to optimise folate status was relatively ineffective and therefore misleading.

There is now a consensus that the preferred public health policy in the prevention of neural tube defects is to fortify food with folic acid.

Choice of Food for Fortification with Folic Acid

Flour, in a variety of forms, is consumed by nearly all people. The range of consumption is not so wide that if flour were fortified with a micronutrient such as folic acid some people would consume almost nothing and others many times the average intake. For this reason, flour in many countries is already fortified with vitamins and minerals. The addition of another vitamin, folic acid, would be practical and build on existing experience. In the US the Food and Drug Administration (FDA) has already required food manufacturers to fortify flour-based food products with folic acid. Under this rule all products derived from grain flour (bread, rolls, cakes, pasta, cornmeal, rice) must be fortified with folic acid. The level of fortification has been set at twice the restitution level, that is, twice the amount of folic acid that would be required to replace the folic acid removed in the milling process. This amounts to 0.14 mg/100 g of flour, the level which on average is expected to increase the intake of folic acid in the US population by about 0.1 mg/day. While the US has taken the lead in accepting the principle, it is widely felt that the level of fortification is too low, with an expected reduction in the risk of a neural tube defect pregnancy of only 18% [Wald et al. 1998a]. The US Centers for Disease Control has persistently recommended a higher level. On the basis of previous experience with the fortification of flour and the precedent set by the FDA, other countries are likely to adopt flour as the vehicle for folic acid fortification, and the level of fortification is likely to be higher in other countries. Canada has already taken the decision to fortify flour at the same level as the US, and New Zealand is to fortify flour at a level of 0.245 mg/100 g of flour [Godfrey Oakley, pers. commun.], which may be expected to reduce the neural tube defect risk by about 40%.

Folate Terminology and the Need to Express Total Folate Intake in Folic Acid Equivalents

The terms folic acid and folate are confusingly used as synonyms. They are not the same. Folic acid is the name for pteroylglutamic acid (PGA). This consists of a double-ringed pteridine portion joined to *p*-aminobenzoic acid (PABA) and glutamic acid. Folic acid is used in vitamin supplementation and food fortification and has four important features: (1) it is oxidised and therefore stable; (2) it has only one glutamic acid residue; (3) it is synthetic and is not present in natural food, and (4) it is about twice as bioavailable as natural folate [Gregory, 1995].

Folate is a generic term that includes folic acid as well as derivatives that have the folic acid structure as their central element. Natural folates are derivatives of folic acid that occur in natural food. They have two important features: (1) they exist in a reduced form by either having two extra hydrogen atoms on the fifth and sixth carbon atoms (dihydrofolate, DHF) or four extra hydrogen atoms on the carbon atoms numbers 5, 6, 7 and 8 (tetrahydrofolate, THF), and (2) they have multiple glutamic acid residues (polyglutamates).

There is an important source of confusion that needs to be avoided. Oxidation of reduced natural folate does not yield the stable oxidised folic acid because the oxidation does not involve removal of the 2 or 4 hydrogen atoms that specifies DHF or THF. The oxidation leads to the molecules splitting at the 9, 10 carbon bond, destroying the molecule and therefore its folic acid activity. Such oxidation readily occurs with natural folate and is the reason that natural folate is unstable and readily destroyed by heat. The nonreduced synthetic folic acid is not subject to this effect and is therefore stable. It is therefore fortunate that the form suitable for food fortification is the stable form.

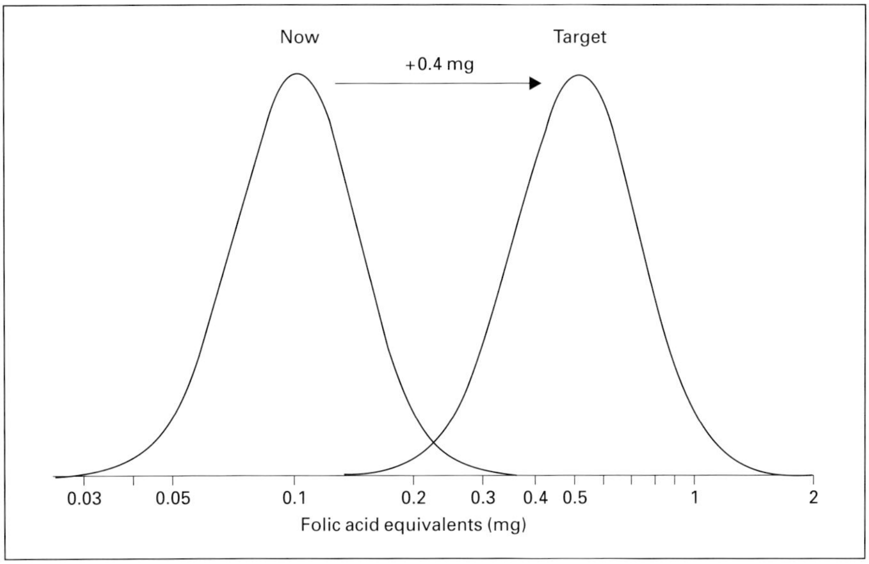

Fig. 2. The shift in the distribution of folate consumption to receive a target of an extra 0.4 mg/day intake expressed in folic acid equivalents.

To avoid confusion in nomenclature it would be helpful if the following definitions were used (1) folate consists of all substances that contain the core molecule folic acid (PGA) whether folic acid itself or its derivatives; (2) folic acid is PGA alone, and (3) natural folate consists of derivatives of PGA that occur naturally in food.

The greater bioavailability of folic acid compared with natural folate is also a fortunate advantage for food fortification, but it means that simply adding folic acid and natural folate in micrograms of intake is somewhat misleading in assessing biologically useful folate intake. To overcome this it is probably best to adopt one of the following three approaches: (1) if the assessment is based on folic acid intake it should be based on intake of synthetic sources (fortification and supplements); (2) if intake is based on natural folate consumption this should exclude the consumption of folic acid from synthetic sources, and (3) if intake is to be assessed on the basis of total folate (folic acid plus natural folate consumption) the combination would be better expressed in folic acid equivalents, in which the intake of natural folates would be halved to allow for their reduced bioavailability relative to folic acid. Figure 2 shows this shift in the distribution of the folate intake expressed in folic acid equivalents to achieve the recommended target increase in daily intake of 0.4 mg of folic acid recommended by many public health authorities for the prevention of neural tube defects.

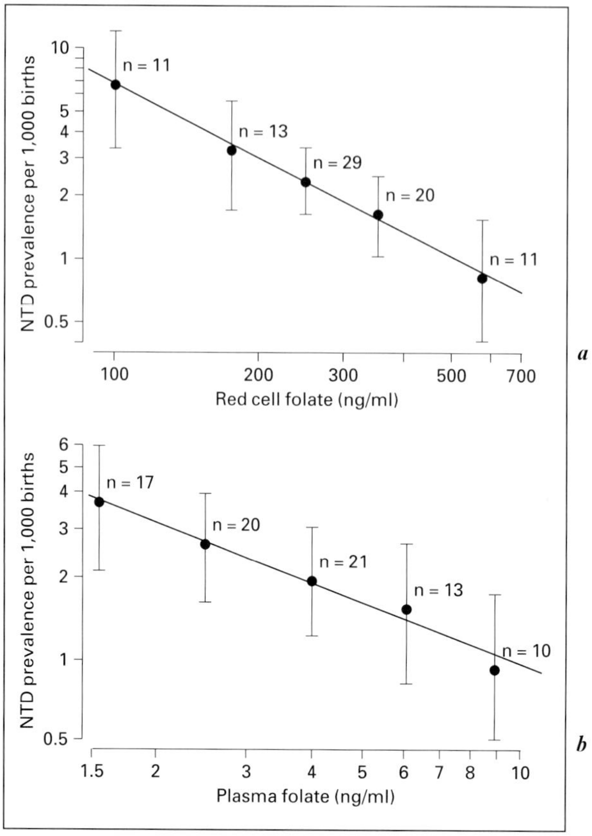

Fig. 3. The relationship between birth prevalence of neural tube defects in the absence of antenatal screening and selective abortion and red cell folate (***a***) and plasma folate (***b***) based on data published by Daly et al. [1995].

Dose-Response Relationship Between Folate Intake and the Risk of Neural Tube Defects

It is recognised that increasing folic acid intake increases plasma and red cell folate levels. From the perspective of neural tube defect prevention, plasma or serum folate levels may be of greater relevance than red cell folate levels, because the embryo obtains folate from the maternal plasma. Plasma folate levels reflect immediate intakes of folates, whereas red cell folate represents folate status over the previous months. When plotted on a log scale, the risk of having a child with a neural tube defect is linearly associated with plasma folate and red cell folate levels in early pregnancy [Daly et al., 1995]. Figure 3

Table 1. Relative risk of having a neural tube defect pregnancy according to maternal plasma folate level

Plasma folate, arbitrary units	Relative neural tube defect risk[1]
1.0	1.00
1.5	0.74
2.0	0.59
2.5	0.50
5.0	0.30
10.0	0.18

[1] log relative risk = –0.7519 × log relative plasma folate level from the relationship in the lower part of figure 3. Wald and Noble [1999], from Daly et al. [1995].

shows the relationship between birth prevalence of neural tube defects and red cell folate or plasma folate taken from the paper by Daly et al. The two graphs show that a proportional increase in red cell or plasma folate level is linearly associated with a proportional decrease in risk. We recently showed how the relationship can be conveniently simplified [Wald et al., 1998a] to:

$$\text{relative odds of a neural tube defect pregnancy} = (\text{new red cell folate/old red cell folate})^{-1.22}$$

The corresponding equation for plasma folate is the same but raised to the power of –0.75 (derived indirectly from an analysis of data presented in table 1 of Daly et al. [1995]). Table 1 shows the relative odds of having a neural tube defect pregnancy according to maternal plasma folate level.

In the recent study by Daly et al. [1997], a 0.4-mg/day folic acid supplement increased the red cell folate level in a sample of women from 311 to 571 ng/ml, a 1.84-fold increase. The predicted relative risk of a neural tube defect pregnancy was therefore $1.84^{-1.22}$ or 0.475, a risk reduction of 0.525 (1–0.475) or 53%. This is exactly the summary risk reduction in the observational studies of vitamins containing folic acid, typically 0.4 mg (table 2). There is therefore striking agreement between the risk estimation based on the data of Daly et al. [1995, 1997] and the observational studies of vitamin supplementation and of neural tube defects [Wald, 1994, 1995]. This validates the dose-response model between blood folate and neural tube defect risk up to doses of about 0.4 mg/day. The MRC Vitamin Study [1991] used a dose of folic acid of 4 mg/day and the median serum folate in the women allocated to folic acid was about 9 times higher than among the controls; the model predicts a relative

Table 2. Observational studies of the use of vitamins containing folic acid and the occurrence of neural tube defects [based on Wald, 1994]

Study	Relative risk (95% confidence interval)
Winship et al. [1984]	0.14 (0.003–1.11)
Mulinare et al. [1988]	0.41 (0.26–0.66)
Mills et al. [1989]	0.94 (0.80–1.10)
Milunsky et al. [1989]	0.29 (0.15–0.55)
Werler et al. [1993]	0.6 (0.4–0.8)
Bower and Stanley [1992]	0.11 (0.01–1.33)
Combined	0.47 (0.29–0.76)

risk of 0.19 ($9^{-0.75}$) which is virtually identical to the relative risk among women not already pregnant at the time of randomisation (relative risk 0.17, 95% confidence interval 0.05–0.59). This offers some validation of the model over a wide range of blood folate levels. What is less clear is the dose-response relationship between folic acid and either red cell or serum folate levels. This needs to be determined by further work. The present data [Truswell and Kounnavong, 1997; Daly et al., 1997; Malinow et al., 1998] are too variable and the estimates are imprecise.

Available evidence therefore shows that an extra 0.4 mg of folic acid daily will increase plasma folate by about 80% and will reduce neural tube defects by about 50%.

The Concept of the Minimum Fully Effective Dose

Increasing folic acid consumption increases blood folate levels which in turn will reduce the risk of neural tube defects. The linear proportional dose-response relationship has not been shown to have a plateau beyond which further increases in folic acid yield no further protective effect. On physiological grounds there is likely to be some such plateau, because above certain levels folic acid is excreted into the urine. The level at which this occurs has not yet been determined. It could be termed the minimum fully effective dose (MFED), because further increases in dose will have no additional protective effect. The term minimum effective dose has been used [Daly et al., 1997] but from a public health perspective it is the minimum dose that can achieve a *full* effect

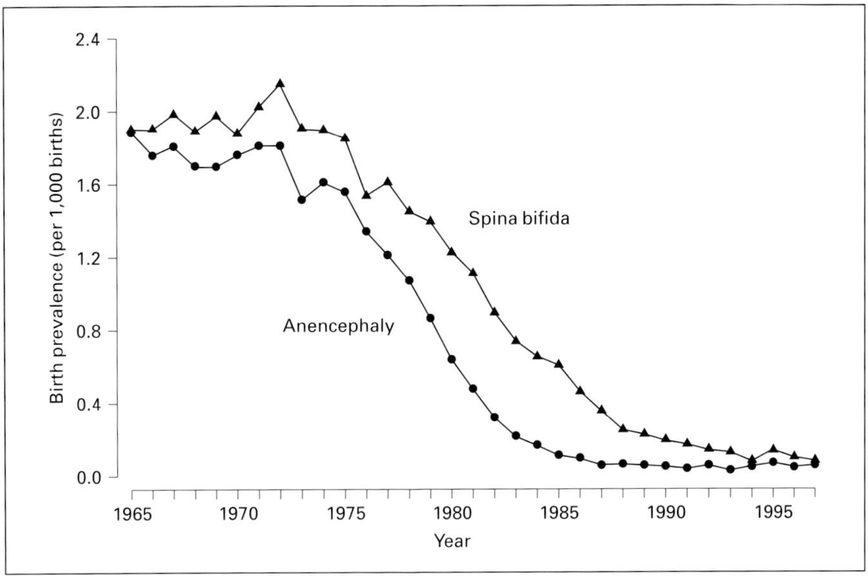

Fig. 4. Prevalence of neural tube defects at birth in England and Wales 1995–1997, based on notifications to the Office of National Statistics adjusted for underascertainment.

that needs to be determined. If there is no reason to believe that this level will be toxic, then it should become the target dose. Public health authorities may not wish to fortify food at levels sufficient to achieve the MFED, for example on grounds of safety, so the target dose may be less than the MFED. At present it would seem reasonable for public health authorities to set a level of fortification capable of achieving an average extra folic acid intake of 0.4 mg/day and revise this in the light of relevant research. Because of the variation in flour intake, some individuals will achieve lower intakes and others will have higher intakes. To specify the distribution of intakes, the 5th and 95th centiles can be specified from modelling studies. The 99th and 1st centiles are likely to be unstable and, respectively, too high and too low because of the error arising from the variation in estimates of intake within the same individual.

Monitoring Trends in the Birth Prevalence of Neural Tube Defects: England and Wales as an Example

In the past, Britain had one of the highest birth prevalences of neural tube defects in the world, and now it has one of the lowest. Figure 4 illustrates the decline in the birth prevalence of neural tube defects and table 3 shows

Table 3. Number of births with anencephaly and spina bifida in England and Wales 1965–1996

Year	Anencephaly	Spina bifida	Total
1965	1,346	1,454	2,800
1970	1,137	1,309	2,446
1975	775	986	1,761
1980	342	712	1,054
1985	59	352	411
1990	26	116	142
1995	35	72	107
1996	24	57	81

Data from notifications of birth defects to OPCS [Rogers and Weatherall, 1976; OPCS, 1983–1986]. Separate data on spina bifida without anencephaly are not published for the period of 1986–1996 but were obtained as a personal communication from Mrs. B. Botting at the Office of National Statistics (formerly the OPCS).

the actual numbers used to construct the figure, which allows for underascertainment. Much of the decline in the birth prevalence of neural tube defects is attributable to antenatal screening and diagnosis and the abortion of affected pregnancies. In countries such as Britain where such screening is common, the main impact on prevention through increasing the consumption of folic acid will be substantial reduction in the number of abortions carried out because of a neural tube defect pregnancy. It would be helpful if national public health agencies monitored the birth prevalence of neural tube defects and, if possible, the contribution of antenatal screening and selective abortion to any changes in the rates.

Homocysteine and the Prevention of Ischaemic Heart Disease

Folic acid supplementation has been shown to reduce average serum homocysteine levels. A recent meta-analysis of randomised controlled trials that assessed the effects of folic acid-based supplements on blood homocysteine concentrations showed that folic acid reduced homocysteine levels by 25% (95% confidence interval; 23–28%, ($p < 0.001$) with similar effects in the range of about 1–5 mg of folic acid daily [Homocysteine Lowering Trialists' Collaboration, 1998]. Homocysteine is associated in retrospective and prospective studies with atherosclerotic disease including ischaemic heart disease [Wald et al., 1998b]. The association is independent of other risk factors. Various genetic abnormalities and variants associated with high homocysteine levels are themselves associated with an increased risk of vascular disease. It is likely that the association between homocysteine and ischaemic heart disease is causal, and it has been estimated that if 0.4 mg folic acid per day on average reduces homocysteine levels by 1.9 μmol/l [Ward et al., 1997], this would be equivalent to a 10% reduction in ischaemic heart disease mortality in Western countries (95% confidence interval; 4–16%) [Wald et al., 1998b]. With a 25% reduction in homocysteine levels (3 μmol/l reduction) the estimated reduction in ischaemic heart disease mortality would be 16%. Although the reduction in ischaemic heart disease mortality achievable through reducing homocysteine levels by consuming folic acid is relatively modest (about 10–15%), because death from ischaemic heart disease is so common it would represent a major public health benefit, avoiding over 10,000 premature deaths from this disease each year in Britain alone.

The Need to Revise RDAs for Folic Acid

Before the recognition of the importance of folic acid deficiency in causing neural tube defects and the effects of folic acid in reducing homocysteine levels that are thought to be involved in the pathogenesis of ischaemic heart disease, there was little reason to specify RDA values for folic acid in excess of 0.2 mg/day. Now the position is quite different. It is essential that these be revised and specified in folic acid equivalents at a level no less than 0.4 mg/day. This will mean reversing a recent trend in lowering RDA in Europe and North America. Without this initiative it will be more difficult for food manufacturers to supply the necessary level of fortification on a voluntary basis in countries where mandatory fortification is not introduced. Such an upward revision has been done in the US; the US National Academy of Sciences, in its report *Dietary Reference Intakes*, recommended that 'while all adult men and women need 400 μg of folate daily, it is crucial that women aged 19–50 years ingest a further 400 μg of folic acid to reduce the risk of having a baby with neural tube defects' [Droste, 1998].

Conclusions

Flour is a suitable foodstuff that can be used as a vehicle for folic acid fortification. Fortification of flour in this way would provide a population strategy for the prevention of neural tube defects that would be effective, economical, and safe. No other public health measure would have as large an effect in the prevention of a serious congenital abnormality and it is possible that it will also have significant impact on the prevention of vascular disease in the community. A level designed to achieve an average increase in intake of folic acid over background folate levels of 0.4 mg/day would be a reasonable target with surveillance designed to assess the distribution of intake with the aim of monitoring the tails of the distributions so that few people eat less than about 0.2 or 0.3 mg and few eat more than about 1.5 mg/day. Current evidence indicates that those in the lower tail of the distribution will benefit from some preventive effect while there is no evidence that those in the upper tail will suffer any untoward effects.

References

Bower C, Stanley FJ: Periconceptional vitamin supplementation and neural tube defects; evidence from a case-control study in Western Australia and a review of recent publications. J Epidemiol Comm Health 1992;46:157–161.

Cuskelly GJ, McNulty H, Scott JM: Effect of increasing dietary folate on red-cell folate: Implications for prevention of neural tube defects. Lancet 1996;347:657–659.

Daly LE, Kirke PN, Molloy AM, Weir DG, Scott JM: Folate levels and neural defects. JAMA 1995;274: 1698–1702.

Daly S, Mills JL, Molloy AM, Conley M, Lee YJ, Kirke PN, Weir DG, Scott JM: Minimum effective dose of folic acid for food fortification to prevent neural tube defects. Lancet 1997;350:1666–1669.

Droste TM: US study recommends daily amount of vitamins. Lancet 1998;351:1113.

Gregory JF III: The bioavailability of folate; in Baily LB (ed): Folate in Health and Disease. New York, Dekker, 1995, pp 195–235.

Homocysteine Lowering Trialists' Collaboration: Lowering blood homocysteine with folic acid-based supplements: Meta-analysis of randomised trials. BMJ 1998;316:894–898.

Malinow MR, Duell PB, Hess DL, Anderson PH, Kruger WD, Phillipson BE, Gluckman RA, Block PC, Upson BM: Reduction of plasma homocysteine levels by breakfast cereal fortified with folic acid in patients with coronary heart disease. N Engl J Med 1998;338:1009–1015.

Mills JL, Rhoads GG, Simpson JL, Cunningham GL, Conley MR, Lassman MR, Walden ME, Depp OR, Hoffman HJ: The absence of a relation between the periconceptional use of vitamins and neural-tube defects. N Engl J Med 1989;321:430–435.

Milunsky A, Jick H, Jick SS, Bruell CL, Maclaughlin DS, Rothman KJ, Willett W: Multivitamin/folic acid supplementation in early pregnancy reduces the prevalence of neural tube defects. JAMA 1989; 262:2847–2852.

MRC Vitamin Study Research Group: Prevention of neural tube defects: Results of the MRC Vitamin Study. Lancet 1991;338:132–137.

Mulinare J, Cordero JF, Erickson D, Berry RJ: Periconceptional use of multivitamins and the occurrence of neural tube defects. JAMA 1988;260:3141–3145.

Office of Population Censuses and Surveys 1983–1986: Congenital Malformations Statistics Series MB3 Nos 1–3.

Office of Population Censuses and Surveys: The Dietary and Nutritional Survey of British Adults. London, HMSO, 1990.

Rogers SC, Weatherall JAC: Anencephalus, spina bifida and congenital hydrocephalus, England and Wales 1964–1972. Office of Population Censuses and Surveys. Studies on Medical and Population Subjects No 32, 1976.

Truswell AS, Kounnavong S: Quantitative responses of serum folate to increasing intakes of folic acid in healthy women. Eur J Clin Nutr 1997;51:839–845.

Wald NJ: Folic acid and neural tube defects: The current evidence and implications for prevention; in Neural Tube Defects. Ciba Found Symp 181. Chichester, Wiley, 1994, pp 192–211.

Wald NJ: Folic acid and the prevention of neural tube defects: The need for public health action. The scientific basis for vitamin intake in human nutrition. Bibl Nutr Dieta. Basel, Karger, 1995, vol 52, pp 56–65.

Wald NJ, Noble J: Primary prevention of neural tube defects; in Rodeck CH, Whittle MJ (eds): Fetal Medicine: Basic Science and Clinical Practice. Churchill Livingstone, London, 1999, pp 283–290.

Wald NJ, Law MR, Jordan R: Folic acid food fortification to prevent neural tube defects. Lancet 1998a; 351:834.

Wald NJ, Watt HC, Law MR, Weir DG, McPartlin J, Scott JM: Homocysteine and ischaemic heart disease: Results of a prospective study with implications on prevention. Arch Intern Med 1998b; 158:862–867.

Ward M, McNulty H, McPartlin JM, Strain JJ, Weir D, Scott JM: Plasma homocysteine, a risk factor for cardiovascular disease, can be effectively lowered by physiological amounts of folic acid. QJ Med 1997;90:519–524.

Werler MM, Shapiro S, Mitchel AA: Periconceptional folic acid exposure and risk of occurrent neural tube defects. JAMA 1993;269:1257–1261.

Winship KA, Cahal DA, Weber JCP, Griffin JP: Maternal drug histories and central nervous system anomalies. Arch Dis Child 1984;59:1052–1060.

Prof. Nicholas J. Wald, St Bartholomew's and the Royal School of Medicine and Dentistry,
Wolfson Institute for Preventive Medicine, Department of Environment & Preventive Medicine,
Charterhouse Square, London EC 1M 6BQ (UK)
Tel. +44 171 982 62 69, Fax +44 171 982 62 70, E-Mail n.j.wald@mds.qmw.ac.uk

Walter P, Hornig D, Moser U (eds): Functions of Vitamins beyond Recommended Dietary Allowances. Bibl Nutr Dieta. Basel, Karger, 2001, No 55, pp 34–41

Rationale for Risk Reduction of Cardiovascular Disease Using Homocysteine Concentration in Blood and Plasma as Biomarker: Support by Clinical Data

Klaus Pietrzik

Institute of Nutritional Science, Department of Pathophysiology of Nutrition, University of Bonn, Germany

The metabolism of a substrate is closely linked to that of its cofactor(s). In the case of the amino acid homocysteine, there are three vitamins acting as cofactors or coenzymes, namely vitamins B_6, B_{12} and folate. Vitamin B_6 in the form of pyridoxal-5-phosphate is involved in the formation of cystathionine from homocysteine (so-called transsulfuration pathway). It is also essential for the formation of 5,10-methylenetetrahydrofolate (5,10-MTHF) from tetrahydrofolate (THF) and is therefore closely related to the metabolism of folate as well. The latter is – together with vitamin B_{12} – involved in the remethylation of homocysteine to methionine. In this reaction, the methyl group of 5-methyl-THF is transported to vitamin B_{12} linked to the enzyme *homocysteine methyltransferase* to yield methylcobalamin enzyme. Finally, this complex adds the methyl group to homocysteine to form methionine.

A number of human as well as animal studies have been conducted to evaluate the role of the mentioned B vitamins in the metabolism of homocysteine. However, these studies differ with regard to the biological situation of the participants upon onset of the study. Four different situations have to be distinguished: (1) Vitamin deficiency and the occurrence of elevated homocysteine concentrations. (2) Treatment of elevated homocysteine concentrations (hyperhomocysteinemia) not due to vitamin deficiency with (high) doses of one or more vitamins involved in homocysteine metabolism. (3) Reduction of 'normal' homocysteine concentrations with the respective vitamin cofactors.

(4) Normal ranges of the vitamins as determinants of the homocysteine concentration.

These different situations will be distinguished when evaluating the role of the vitamins B_6, B_{12} and folate as determinants of the homocysteine concentration:

(1) In case of deficiency of one or more vitamins involved in homocysteine metabolism, the concentration of this amino acid in plasma is elevated well above of what is observed in the healthy population (5–15 μmol/l). In chronic alcoholics, e.g., homocysteine concentrations were twice as high as in healthy persons. At the same time, pyridoxal-5-phosphate and red blood cell folate concentrations were significantly diminished in alcoholics, whereas vitamin B_{12} was elevated [1]. Since both folate and vitamin B_6 were diminished in alcoholics, it was not possible to estimate if deficiency of both or only one may have led to the elevated homocysteine concentrations. However, others have shown that vitamin B_6 deficiency does not necessarily result in elevated homocysteine concentrations and thus is not a good indicator of vitamin B_6 status [2]. In case of severe cobalamin or folate deficiency, homocysteine in plasma may reach as high concentrations as observed with genetic disorders of homocysteine metabolism, e.g. dysfunction of the enzyme *cystathionine-β synthase*. The high concentrations may be explained by an increased influx of homocysteine from the cells into the extracellular compartment including plasma, rather than by a diminished clearance from the plasma through *homocysteine methyltransferase* [3]. After vitamin treatment, these homocysteine concentrations rapidly return to normal ranges [4].

(2) Treatment of hyperhomocysteinemia routinely includes supplementation with pharmacological doses of one or more of the relevant B vitamins. In the case of *cystathionine-β-synthase* deficiency, enzyme activity is effectively enhanced by treatment with large doses of vitamin B_6 [5]. Others have used a combination of all three relevant cofactors to treat milder forms of homocysteinemia [6, 7]. This multivitamin supplementation clearly resulted in a 50% reduction of plasma homocysteine concentrations, but given alone, only folate was able to induce similar reductions in this group, whereas vitamin B_{12} was little effective and vitamin B_6 failed to show an effect.

(3) When healthy individuals with homocysteine concentrations in the normal range are supplemented with the respective vitamin cofactors, they still show a significant reduction of this atherogenic amino acid. Depending on the pretreatment on the homocysteine concentration and on the dose and combination of vitamins used, this effect can be as much as 10–20%. We supplemented young women (21–31 years of age) with a combination of folic acid (400 μg), vitamin B_{12} (6 μg) and vitamin B_6 (2 mg) daily for 12 weeks. Already after 4 weeks the homocysteine concentration was significantly

reduced by 17%. Thereafter, no further decrease was observed. When given to a different age group, namely men and women of middle age (40–65 years), this vitamin combination led to a 11% reduction of the homocysteine plasma concentration after supplementation for 4 weeks. However, pretreatment levels were higher than in the younger group, i.e. a mean of 10.0 μmol/l in the middle-aged group versus 8.0 μmol/l in the young women. Others have shown even more substantial reductions of homocysteine (up to –37%), but high (pharmacological) doses of the vitamins in combination were given [8] or other routes of supplementation than peroral ingestion were chosen [9].

Since the assessment of vitamin nutritional status by the measurement of plasma concentrations may be subject to both analytical error and biologically defined confounding factors, it may also be worth looking at a functional parameter of vitamin status. Homocysteine is such a functional parameter. Thus, the above findings of a significant reduction of homocysteine concentrations in healthy people with a vitamin status currently regarded as adequate may be an indicator of a suboptimal vitamin status. However, it could be argued that supplementation of a cofactor will, to some extent, always lead to an enhancement of enzyme activity and as such to the reduction of substrate levels. Subsequently, it might be more relevant to look at the association of vitamin and homocysteine concentrations *before* the onset of treatment (in this case vitamin supplementation).

(4) Figure 1 shows the relationship between homocysteine and plasma folate concentrations of the age groups that participated in the supplementation studies of young women and middle-aged men and women. It can be seen that homocysteine concentrations increase as plasma folate concentrations decrease. This is less pronounced with folate concentrations in the range of about 20–65 nmol/l but more pronounced with folate concentrations below that range. The association between plasma folate and homocysteine is statistically significant and is best described by an inverse regression ($r=0.55$, $p<0.001$). When looking at red blood cell folate and homocysteine, this relationship is similar even though it is less strong (fig. 2, $r=0.32$, $p<0.001$).

Vitamins B_{12} and B_6 do not seem to be associated with homocysteine, as no significant relationship was observed in our study populations (values not shown). This lack of a role of vitamin B_6 as determinant of homocysteine status is in line with results of the literature [2, 6, 7]. It also confirms own results from a supplementation study with vitamin B_6 alone versus supplementation with folate alone or in combination with vitamin B_6 [10]. Thus, vitamin B_6 does not seem to be a determinant of homocysteine status, at least not in healthy individuals of the age we looked at. Results from 1,160 adult survivors of the original Framingham cohort seem to contradict this statement.

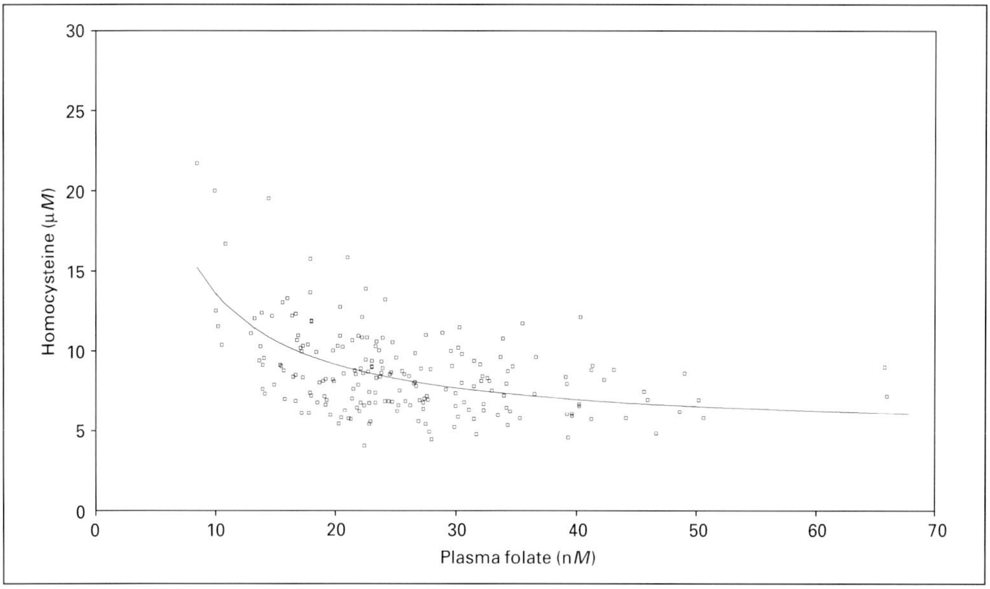

Fig. 1. Relationship between homocysteine and plasma folate in unsupplemented men and women, n = 201 (r = 0.55, p < 0.001).

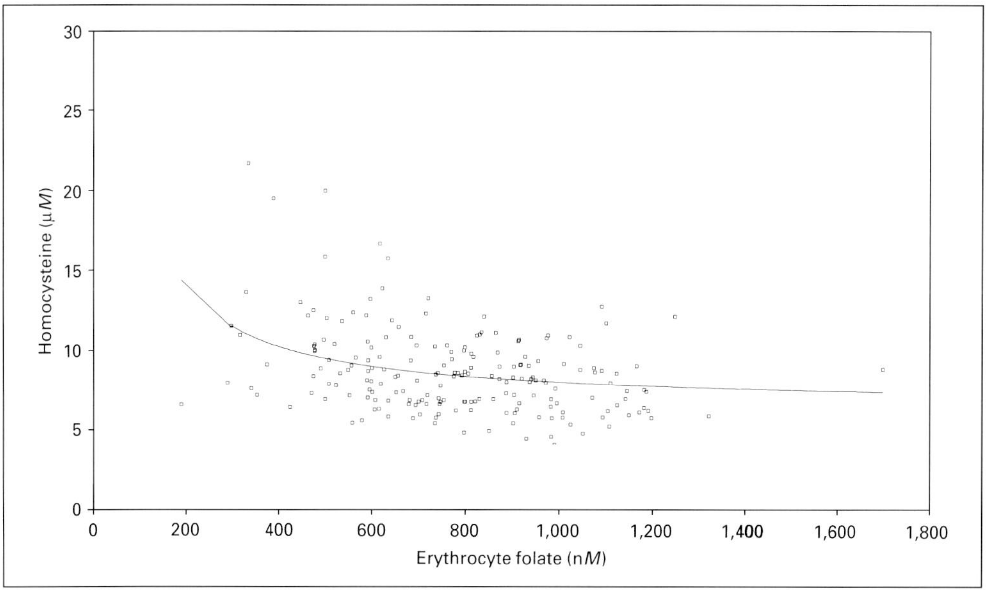

Fig. 2. Relationship between homocysteine and red blood cell folate in unsupplemented men and women, n = 201 (r = 0.32, p < 0.001).

Selhub et al. [11] found an inverse association of homocysteine and plasma vitamin B_6 as well as vitamin B_6 intake. The observed association was mainly due to the occurrence of very low vitamin B_6 concentrations in the lowest decile compared to the mean vitamin B_6 concentration in the highest decile. However, it is questionable if the vitamin concentrations in the lowest decile (about 15 nmol/l) can still be considered adequate (and as such would contradict our statement) or rather are an indicator of a suboptimal vitamin status or even of a vitamin B_6 deficiency.

The role of vitamin B_{12} as determinant of homocysteine status in healthy individuals remains unclear. We could not confirm the findings of Pancharuniti et al. [12] of a significant inverse correlation of homocysteine and vitamin B_{12} in healthy men even though vitamin concentrations were comparable to those of our study participants. Selhub et al. [11] found weak associations between homocysteine and vitamin B_{12} plasma concentrations. However, subjects in the lowest vitamin B_{12} decile had a mean concentration of only 100 pmol/l. As elderly persons (participants of the Framingham Study ranged from 67 to 96 years of age) often develop vitamin B_{12} deficiency because of atrophic gastritis, vitamin B_{12} plasma concentrations might be useful as determinants of homocysteine in this age group. However, speaking of 'healthy' individuals, vitamin B_{12} seems to play a minor role as determinant of the plasma homocysteine concentration. It might also be possible that different analytical techniques result in different concentrations of the respective vitamins. This would lead to lack of comparability of the 'true' biological vitamin plasma concentration of the subjects in our study and those mentioned above and may be an explanation for the differences observed.

Summarizing the role of vitamins B_{12}, B_6 and folate, the latter seems to play the most important role as determinant of the homocysteine plasma concentration in healthy individuals up to the age of 60 years.

Currently, plasma folate concentrations >7–8 nmol/l and red blood cell folate concentrations >500 nmol/l are regarded as sufficient. These values have been defined on the basis of the absence of clinical signs of folate deficiency (megaloblastic anemia, leukopenia, thrombopenia) as well as morphological alterations of blood cells (increased lobe average of neutrophil granulocytes) indicating an early stage of folate deficiency [13, 14]. However, these blood concentrations do not seem to be sufficient when looking at a functional parameter of folate status, i.e. homocysteine. Figures 1 and 2 show that the homocysteine concentration strongly increases with plasma folate concentrations ca. <20 nmol/l and erythrocyte concentrations <500–600 nmol/l. Even though exact threshold values cannot be derived from these regression curves, the discrepancy between the currently accepted plasma threshold levels of 7–8 nmol/l and those of 20–25 nmol/l derived from utilizing homocysteine as a functional parameter of folate status becomes obvious.

To influence and to optimize this established risk factor of atherosclerosis from early age on, it may be necessary to increase the folate plasma (and red blood cell) concentrations. Current German RDA levels suggest a folate intake of 300 μg folate for adults. US recommended dietary allowances are 400 μg dietary folate for adults. The US RDAs have been reformulated recently [15] on the basis of data from studies having included homocysteine in evaluating the adequacy of folate nutritional status [16, 17]. Jacob et al. [17] conducted a 'depletion-repletion' study in adult men and determined plasma homocysteine as an index of functional folate deficiency in response to graded intakes of folate. After consuming a low folate diet for 30 days, a moderate folate deficiency was observed; concomitantly, plasma homocysteine was increased significantly. During the folate repletion periods, about 84% of the former US RDA of 200 μg dietary folate was fed which was sufficient to increase plasma folate concentrations; however, the high homocysteine concentrations were not restored to pre-depletion values. In contrast, an amount of 440 μg dietary folate/day resulted in a clear decrease of the elevated homocysteine concentrations in that study.

O'Keefe et al. [16] present additional support for the inadequacy of the former dietary folate allowances. Healthy women with adequate folate stores received 200 μg folate/day for 70 days which resulted in (dramatic) decreases of serum and red blood cell folate concentrations. Homocysteine changed inversely with clear evidence of elevated concentrations and a 50% higher mean compared to women receiving 300 or 400 μg folate/day. Homocysteine concentrations of the latter groups were comparable at the end of the study. However, serum folate concentrations differed significantly among these groups; up to 7.5 nmol/l were obtained with a folate intake of 300 μg folate/day for 70 days, whereas a mean concentration of 14 μmol/l was observed with a folate intake of 400 μg/day.

These data aim to show that the former US and current German RDA for folate are probably (far) too low to meet functional folate demands and to obtain optimal homocysteine concentrations. Thus, to influence this strong risk factor for atherosclerotic diseases, the German and other European dietary intake recommendations of folate should be reformulated.

Conclusion

The metabolism of a substrate is closely linked to that of its cofactor(s). In the case of homocysteine, vitamins B_{12}, B_6 and folate are involved in its metabolism. To evaluate the role of these vitamins as determinants of homocysteine concentration in the *healthy* population, only results from this group were considered.

In the healthy population with 'normal' homocysteine concentrations and a vitamin status currently regarded as adequate, folate seems to play the most important role in determining the plasma homocysteine concentration. This has been derived from supplementation studies as well as from statistical correlation analysis regarding the relationship of these three vitamins to homocysteine.

Until now, recommended dietary allowances for folate have been defined on the basis of the absence of clinical signs of deficiency as well as of morphological alterations of blood cells indicating an early stage of folate deficiency. However, these RDA values do not seem to be sufficient when looking at homocysteine as a functional parameter of folate status. Due to the important role of the folate status as determinant of the homocysteine concentration, it may be necessary to newly define an adequate folate concentration and to reassess the dietary allowances for this B vitamin.

References

1 Cravo ML, Gloria LM, Selhub J, Nadeau MR, Camilo ME, Resende MP, Cardoso JN, Leitno CN, Mira FC: Hyperhomocysteinemia in chronic alcoholism: Correlation with folate, vitamin B_{12}, and vitamin B_6 status. Am J Clin Nutr 1996;63:220–224.

2 Miller JW, Ribaya-Mercado JD, Russell RM, Shepard DC, Morrow FD, Cochary EF, Sadowski JA, Gershoff SN, Selhub J: Effect of vitamin B_6 deficiency on fasting plasma homocysteine concentrations. Am J Clin Nutr 1992;55:1154–1160.

3 Guttormsen AB, Schneede J, Ueland PM, Refsum H: Kinetics of total plasma homocysteine in subjects with hyperhomocysteinemia due to folate or cobalamin deficiency. Am J Clin Nutr 1996; 63:194–202.

4 Stabler SP, Lindenbaum J, Allen RH: The use of homocysteine and other metabolites in the specific diagnosis of vitamin B_{12} deficiency. J Nutr 1996;126:1266S–1272S.

5 Perry TL, Hansen S, Love DL, Crawford LE: Treatment of homocysteinuria with a low-methionine diet, supplemental cysteine, and a methyl donor. Lancet 1968;ii:474–478.

6 Ubbink JB, van der Merwe A, Vermaak WJH, Delport R: Hyperhomocysteinemia and the response to vitamin supplementation. Clin Invest 1993;71:993–998.

7 Ubbink JB, Vermaak WJH, van der Merwe A, Becker PJ, Delport R, Potgieter HC: Vitamin requirements for the treatment of hyperhomocysteinemia in humans. J Nutr 1994;124:1927–1933.

8 Ubbink JB, Becker PJ, Vermaak WJH, Delport R: Results of B-vitamin supplementation study used in a prediction model to define a reference range for plasma homocysteine. Clin Chem 1995; 41:1033–1037.

9 Naurath HJ, Joosten E, Riezler R, Stabler SP, Allen RH, Lindenbaum J: Effects of vitamin B_{12}, folate, and vitamin B_6 supplements in elderly people with normal serum vitamin concentrations. Lancet 1995;346:85–89.

10 Dierkes J: Vitamin requirements for the reduction of homocysteine blood levels in healthy young women; thesis, Bonn 1994.

11 Selhub J, Jacques PF, Wilson PWF, Rush D, Rosenberg IH: Vitamin status and intake as primary determinants of homocysteinemia in an elderly population. JAMA 1993;270:2693–2698.

12 Pancharuniti N, Lewis CA, Sauberlich HE, Perkins LL, Go RCP, Alvarez JO, Macaluso M, Acton RT, Copeland RB, Cousins AL, Gore TB, Cornwell PE, Roseman JM: Plasma homocyst(e)ine, folate, and vitamin B_{12} concentrations and risk for early-onset coronary artery disease. Am J Clin Nutr 1994;59:940–948.
13 Hages M, Pietrzik K: Untersuchungen zur Bewertung der Folatversorgung bei Kindern unter Berücksichtigung des Cobalamin- und Eisenhaushalts. 1. Mitteilung: Veränderungen im Differenzialblutbild in Abhängigkeit von den Vitamin- und Ferritinkonzentrationen in Serum bzw. Erythrozyten. Int J Vitam Nutr Res 1985;55:59–67.
14 Pietrzik K: Folate deficiency: Morphological and functional consequences. Bibl Nutr Dieta. Basel, Karger, 1989, vol 44, pp 123–130.
15 Dietary Reference Intakes: Thiamin, Riboflavin, Niacin, Vitamin B_6, Folate, Vitamin B_{12}, Pantothenic Acid, Biotine and Choline. Prepublication Copy. Washington, National Academy of Sciences, 1998.
16 O'Keefe CA, Bailey LB, Thomas EA, Hofler SA, Davis BA, Cerda JJ, Gregory JF III: Controlled dietary folate affects folate status in no pregnant women. J Nutr 1995;125:2717–2725.
17 Jacob RA, Wu MM, Henning SM, Swendseid ME: Homocysteine increases as folate decreases in plasma of healthy men during short-term dietary folate and methyl group restriction. J Nutr 1994; 124:1072–1080.

Prof. Klaus Pietrzik, Institut für Ernährungswissenschaft, Universität Bonn,
D–53115 Bonn (Germany)
Tel. +49 228 73 3753, Fax +49 228 69 2055, E-Mail k.pietrzik@uni.bonn.de

Walter P, Hornig D, Moser U (eds): Functions of Vitamins beyond Recommended Dietary Allowances. Bibl Nutr Dieta. Basel, Karger, 2001, No 55, pp 42–45

Folate and Vitamin B_6 from Diet and Supplements in Relation to Risk of Coronary Heart Disease among Women

Eric B. Rimm

Departments of Epidemiology and Nutrition, Harvard School of Public Health, and Channing Laboratory, Department of Medicine, Brigham and Women's Hospital and Harvard Medical School, Boston, Mass., USA

Three decades ago, premature vascular occlusive disease was identified in patients with inborn metabolic disorders associated with homocysteinuria, leading to the hypothesis that elevated blood homocysteine levels may cause coronary disease [1–3]. More recently, evidence linking moderately elevated blood homocysteine levels to increased risk [4] has focused attention on genetic and lifestyle determinants of homocysteine levels; folate and vitamin B_6 are two important dietary factors which have been shown to influence homocysteine levels [4–8]. Therefore, we examined the relation of intakes of folate and vitamin B_6 to risk of coronary heart disease (CHD) among 80,082 women free of previously diagnosed CHD, diabetes and hypercholesterolemina and followed prospectively for 14 years (1980–1994).

We defined the primary outcome of CHD as documented symptomatic nonfatal myocardial infarction (MI) or fatal CHD occurring after the return of the 1980 questionnaire but before June 1, 1994. We derived average daily intake of folate and vitamin B_6 from a previously validated self-administered food frequency questionnaire [9, 10]. Detailed information on dietary and supplemental sources of these vitamins was incorporated into the intake scores. All nutrients were energy-adjusted using the residual method [10, 11].

During 14 years of follow-up, we identified 658 incident cases of nonfatal MI and 281 cases of fatal CHD. Based on the assessment of average diet, the largest contributors (in absolute percentage) to the overall intake of folate were multiple vitamins (26%), cold cereal (8%), orange juice (8%), lettuce (7.5%), eggs (3%), broccoli (2.5%), and spinach (2%).

The age-adjusted relative risk of CHD was 0.53 (95% CI 0.43, 0.65) comparing women in the highest and lowest quintiles. In multivariate models of folate and CHD, smoking and use of vitamin E supplements were the strongest confounders. The relative risk for folate was 0.61 (95% CI 0.49, 0.75) after adding smoking to the model and was further attenuated to 0.69 (95% CI 0.55, 0.87) after controlling for current use of vitamin E supplements and for other cardiovascular risk factors. In more detailed analyses a diet high in folate from food or supplements conferred a reduction in risk of CHD (for food RR=0.78; 95% CI 0.61, 1.01; quintile 5 – median 379 μg/day versus quintile 1 – median 151 μg/day; for supplements RR=0.76; 95% CI 0.59, 0.98; 400–1000 μg vs no supplements).

We conducted similar analyses for vitamin B_6. As with folate, vitamin supplements were by far the largest contributor to total vitamin B_6 intake. Among the 66.3% of women not taking a multiple vitamin or other supplements containing vitamin B_6, the leading contributors to intake were beef (14%), cold breakfast cereal (9%), potatoes (9%), bananas (8.5%), chicken (7%), milk (5%) and tuna fish (3.5%). Compared to women in the lowest quintile of vitamin B_6 intake, the age-adjusted relative risk of CHD was 0.49 (95% CI 0.40, 0.61) among women in the highest quintile. After controlling for other CHD risk factors the multivariate relative risk was RR=0.67 (95% CI 0.53, 0.85). The multivariate relative risks for folate and vitamin B_6 were not appreciably altered after further controlling for intake of carotene, magnesium, iron, or monounsaturated fat.

Intakes of folate and vitamin B_6 were highly correlated (Spearman r=0.77) and thus, we did not mutually control for both vitamins in a multivariate model. However, among women in the highest quintile of both total folate and total vitamin B_6 compared with women in the lowest quintile of both nutrients the multivariate RR of CHD was 0.55 (95% CI 0.41, 0.74). The relative risk was similar (RR=0.51; 95% CI 0.33, 0.77) after excluding women with supplemental intake of either micronutrient during the follow-up period.

In subanalyses, we examined combinations of factors that may influence folate or homocysteine levels. The inverse relation between folate intake and risk of CHD was stronger among women consuming up to one drink per day (RR=0.69; 95% CI 0.49, 0.97) or greater than one drink per day (RR=0.27; 95% CI 0.13, 0.58) than among women who abstained from alcohol.

In summary, in this population of women, higher intakes of folate from food or supplements, alone or in combination with vitamin B_6, were associated with substantially lower risk of CHD. The lowest risk was among women with intake of folate >400 μg/day and vitamin B_6 >3 mg/day. Our results corroborate and extend recent studies [12–16] showing lower risk of coronary disease in individuals with higher plasma folate and plasma vitamin B_6. Our results suggest that any widespread increase in folate intake will have a favorable impact on CHD rates, but that maximum benefit would be achieved at folate intake of at least 400 μg/day.

Acknowledgement

Supported by Research Grants HL 34594 and CA 40356 from the National Institutes of Health.

References

1 Rimm EB, Willett WC, Hu FB, Sampson L, Colditz GA, Manson JE, Hennekens C, Stampfer MJ: Folate and vitamin B_6 from diet and supplements in relation to risk of coronary heart disease among women. JAMA 1998;279:359–364.
2 McCully KS: Vascular pathology of homocysteinemia: Implications for pathogenesis of arteriosclerosis. Am J Pathol 1969;56:111–128.
3 Mudd SH, Finkelstein JD, Irreverre F, Laster L: Homocystinuria: An enzymatic defect. Science 1964;143:1443–1445.
4 Boushey CJ, Beresford SAA, Omenn GS, Motulsky AG: A quantitative assessment of plasma homocysteine as a risk factor for vascular disease: Probable benefits of increasing folic acid intakes. JAMA 1995;274:1049–1057.
5 Brattstrom LE, Israelsson B, Jeppsson JO, Hultberg BL: Folic acid: An innocuous means to reduce plasma homocyst(e)ine. Scand J Clin Lab Invest 1988;48:215–221.
6 Jacob RA, Wu M, Henning SM, Swendseid ME: Homocysteine increases as folate decreases in plasma of healthy men during short-term dietary folate and methyl group restriction. J Nutr 1994;124:1072–1080.
7 O'Keefe CA, Bailey LB, Thomas EA, Hofler SA, Davis BA, Cerda JJ, Gregory JF III: Controlled dietary folate affects folate status in nonpregnant women. J Nutr 1995;125:2717–2725.
8 Ubbink JB, Vermaak WJH, van der Merwe A, Becker PJ, Delport R, Potgieter HC: Vitamin requirements for the treatment of hyperhomocysteinemia in humans. J Nutr 1994;124:1927–1933.
9 Willett WC, Sampson L, Stampfer MJ, Rosner B, Bain C, Witschi J, Hennekens CH, Speizer FE: Reproducibility and validity of a semiquantitative food frequency questionnaire. Am J Epidemiol 1985;122:51–65.
10 Willett WC: Nutritional Epidemiology. New York, Oxford University Press, 1990.
11 Willett WC, Stampfer MJ: Total energy intake: Implications for epidemiologic analyses. Am J Epidemiol 1986;124:17–27.
12 Verhoef P, Stampfer MJ, Buring JE, Gaziano JM, Allen RH, Stabler SP, Reynolds RD, Kok FJ, Hennekens CH, Willett WC: Homocysteine metabolism and risk of myocardial infarction: Relation with vitamins B_6, B_{12}, and folate. Am J Epidemiol 1996;143:845–859.
13 Chasan-Taber L, Selhub J, Rosenberg IH, Malinow MR, Terry P, Tishler RV, Willett WC, Hennekens CH, Stampfer MJ: A prospective study of folate and vitamin B_6 and risk of myocardial infarction in US physicians. Am Coll Nutr 1996;15:136–143.

14 Morrison HI, Schaubel D, Desmeules M, Wigle DT: Serum folate and risk of fatal coronary heart disease. JAMA 1996;275:1893–1896.
15 Pancharuniti N, Lewis CA, Sauberlich HE, Perkins LL, Go RC, Alvarez JO, Macaluso M, Acton RT, Copeland RB, Cousins AL: Plasma homocyst(e)ine, folate, and vitamin B_{12} concentrations and risk for early-onset coronary artery disease. Am J Clin Nutr 1994;59:940–948.
16 Robinson D, Arheart K, Refsum H, Brattstrom L, Boers G, Ueland P, Rubba P, Palma-Reis R, Meleady R, Daly L, Witteman J, Graham I, for the European COMAC Group. Low circulating folate and vitamin B_6 concentrations: Risk factors for stroke, peripheral vascular disease, and coronary artery disease. Circulation 1998;97:437–443.

Eric B. Rimm, Department of Nutrition, Harvard School of Public Health,
665 Huntington Avenue, Boston, MA 02115 (USA)
Tel. +1 617 432 1843, Fax +1 617 432 2435, E-Mail eric.rimm@channing.harvard.edu

Walter P, Hornig D, Moser U (eds): Functions of Vitamins beyond Recommended Dietary Allowances. Bibl Nutr Dieta. Basel, Karger, 2001, No 55, pp 46–67

Antioxidant Vitamins: Evidence from Biomarkers in Humans

Balz Frei, Mark R. McCall

Linus Pauling Institute, Oregon State University, Corvallis, Oreg., USA

Introduction

Oxidative stress is generally thought to play an important contributory role in the pathogenesis of degenerative diseases, such as atherosclerosis and cancer. Although there are many determinants in the development of these diseases, considerable experimental evidence links the production of reactive oxygen species (ROS) to biological damage that potentially provides mechanistic explanations for the initiation and/or progression of the diseases in question [1–3]. ROS are capable of chemically altering virtually all major classes of biomolecules (e.g. lipids, proteins, DNA) with concomitant changes in structure and function. Human beings, along with other aerobic organisms, have evolved a variety of mechanisms to protect themselves from the potentially deleterious effects of ROS. These include enzymes (e.g. repair enzymes, catalase, superoxide dismutase and glutathione peroxidase) as well as water and lipid-soluble antioxidants such as ascorbate (vitamin C) and α-tocopherol (vitamin E) [2, 3]. Thus, it is generally thought that oxidative pathology results when the production of ROS and ROS products exceeds the cell's capacity to protect or repair itself.

If oxidative damage is an important etiologic factor in the pathogenesis of atherosclerosis and cancer, then it follows that the antioxidant vitamins C and E may play some role in the prevention and/or amelioration of these diseases. Although both vitamins are capable antioxidants in vitro, there is only a limited number of studies in humans that have addressed the efficacy of these vitamins as antioxidants in vivo. One of the major limitations in conducting these studies is that many of the methods developed to assess oxidative damage in in vitro systems (e.g. isolated cells in culture where sample collection and experimental conditions can be rigorously controlled) are not applicable to in vivo studies in human beings. Since in vivo oxidative damage is likely to occur at only a few sites or tissues at any given time, and since products of oxidation are subject to detoxification and metabolism, a suitable biomarker of oxidative damage must be present in sufficiently high concentrations and in accessible tissues to enable collection and quantification. In addition, biomarkers must be sufficiently stable so that they do not degrade or generate additional oxidation products when handled or stored [4]. As might be expected considering these caveats, there are relatively few reliable markers of in vivo oxidative damage. In fact, most of these biomarkers have only recently been developed and their validity remains to be fully established. Markers of oxidative damage occurring in vivo can be classified into three major groups: markers of oxidative damage to lipids, protein and DNA.

Markers of Oxidative Damage to Lipids

Oxidation of membrane and lipoprotein lipids is generally thought to precede, and to some extent mediate, membrane and cellular modifications that have been linked to the initiation and progression of atherosclerosis and cancer [1, 3, 5]. In humans lipid peroxidation is thought to proceed by radical mediated extraction of a hydrogen atom from a methylene carbon on a polyunsaturated fatty acid (PUFA) or a PUFA side chain. The resulting carbon-centered radical may then undergo molecular rearrangement followed by interaction with O_2 to form a peroxyl radical. Among possible fates of the nascent peroxyl radical is the abstraction of a hydrogen atom from an adjacent PUFA side chain, thereby propagating the oxidative injury [1]. Once formed, lipid hydroperoxides can decompose into a variety of breakdown products, some of which are reported to possess cytotoxic, mutagenic and genotoxic properties [6]. Thus, the formation of lipid hydroperoxides and lipid hydroperoxide breakdown products are important events that can be used to monitor the extent of oxidative damage to lipids [1].

The major initial reaction products of PUFA peroxidation are lipid hydroperoxides. Estimates of PUFA peroxidation, therefore, can be obtained by measuring the disappearance of PUFA, formation of lipid hydroperoxides or formation of conjugated double bond systems (i.e. conjugated dienes) that reflect propagation of the initial oxidative injury [1]. These indices of PUFA peroxidation have been extensively used in in vitro studies, however, their use is limited in complex biological systems due to interfering substances and lability in storage.

Lipid oxidative damage in humans has been assessed traditionally by the measurement of thiobarbituric acid-reactive substances (TBARS assay), which are thought to reflect the production of malondialdehyde (MDA), a nonlipophilic peroxidation product of PUFAs containing three or more methylene interrupted double bonds (e.g. arachidonic acid) [1]. Much has been written concerning the lack of specificity of this assay [4, 7, 8], however, it is still widely used due to the fact that the assay is easy to perform and inexpensive. The actual measurement of the TBA-MDA adduct by high-performance liquid chromatography (HPLC) methods increases the specificity of the assay, however, this does not alleviate problems associated with the conditions used in forming the TBA-MDA adduct [8].

Studies that have used the TBARS assay in plasma or urine have in general supported the hypothesis that an imbalance in pro-oxidant/antioxidant status results in lipid damage that potentially contributes to the development of atherosclerosis and cancer [9–13]. Most of these studies have been conducted in smokers, since smoking is thought to be an oxidative stress. Of the studies shown in table 1, those in which the diets of smokers were supplemented with vitamin E (280–600 IU/day) or vitamin C (1,000 mg/day) showed significant reductions in TBARS compared to baseline or unsupplemented control subjects [9, 10, 12]. Nonsmokers were more variable in their responses to supplementation with antioxidant vitamins; only the study of Brown et al. [10] showed a significant reduction in TBARS, compared to control, when the diets of nonsmokers were supplemented with 280 mg/day of vitamin E. Three other studies failed to show an effect of either vitamin C (1,000 mg/day) or vitamin E (100 or 600 IU/day) on TBARS levels in urine or plasma in nonsmokers [11–13]. Taken together, these data suggest that antioxidant vitamin supplementation may be beneficial to subjects exposed to chronic oxidative stress in the form of cigarette smoke.

Breakdown of lipid hydroperoxides results in the generation of aldehydes other than MDA. Of these secondary lipid peroxidation products the α, β unsaturated aldehyde 4-hydroxynonenal (HNE) has gained some limited acceptance as an index of lipid peroxidation [7]. Quantifying HNE as well as other specific aldehyde PUFA breakdown products is technically difficult and as a result their use as biomarkers has been limited. In addition, aldehydes are not specific for lipid peroxidation because they are also formed, for example, by glycoxidation and the reaction of ROS with hydroxy-amino acids.

Aldehydes such as HNE and MDA are immunogenic, thus, in the future antisera and monoclonal antibodies recognizing epitopes of aldehyde adducts on plasma and tissue proteins may prove to be useful markers of lipid and protein oxidation. It has already been shown that antibodies prepared against MDA- and HNE-modified proteins recognize oxidized LDL and other oxidized proteins in atherosclerotic lesions [7, 14]. In addition, in human beings autoantibodies to epitopes on LDL recognize MDA-modified protein [7].

More recently, quantification of F_2-isoprostanes has been suggested as a reliable index of in vivo free radical generation and lipid oxidative damage [15, 16]. F_2-isoprostanes are isomers of prostaglandin F_2 (PGF_2) and have been shown to be products of free radical mediated, cyclooxygenase-independent peroxidation of arachidonic acid. Of the F_2-isoprostanes formed in vivo, 8-*epi*$PGF_{2\alpha}$ has been the most intensively studied. This relatively stable end-product of lipid peroxidation possesses prostaglandin-like biological activity, promoting vasoconstriction [16] and acting as a smooth muscle cell mitogen [17]. Urinary excretion of F_2-isoprostanes and/or 8-*epi*$PGF_{2\alpha}$ has been shown to increase in both humans and animals in diverse settings in which ROS are thought to promote tissue injury [15, 18]. Moreover, measurement of F_2-isoprostanes or 8-*epi*$PGF_{2\alpha}$ correlate well with other measures of lipid peroxidation (e.g. TBARS and lipid hydroperoxides) in in vitro systems (e.g. ex vivo copper-mediated oxidation of LDL) [19]. Interestingly, the assumption that F_2-isoprostane biosynthesis in vivo reflects non-enzymatic arachidonic acid peroxidation has recently been challenged. In both activated platelets [20] and monocytes [21] 8-*epi*$PGF_{2\alpha}$ can be produced by cyclooxygenase-dependent pathways. The relative importance of these enzymatic pathways to the total urinary excretion of 8-*epi* $PGF_{2\alpha}$ appears quite small in vivo, however, use of 8-*epi*$PGF_{2\alpha}$ (as well as the more general measure of F_2-isoprostanes) requires further validation.

Recently, Reilly et al. [22] examined the levels of urinary 8-*epi*$PGF_{2\alpha}$ in chronic cigarette smokers before and after short-term therapy with vitamins C and E. Moderate smokers (15–30 cigarettes/day) were given 100 IU/day of vitamin E for 5 days; heavy smokers were given either 800 IU/day of vitamin E, 2,000 mg/day of vitamin C or a combination of the two vitamins for 5 days. Supplementation of low (100 IU) or high (800 IU) dose vitamin E failed to reduce urinary 8-*epi*$PGF_{2\alpha}$ excretion. In contrast, urinary excretion of 8-*epi*$PGF_{2\alpha}$ was significantly ($p < 0.05$) reduced following therapy with vitamin C alone or in combination with vitamin E. Taken together with the observation that treatment with aspirin, an inhibitor of cyclooxygenase, failed to suppress 8-*epi*$PGF_{2\alpha}$ production [22], these data provide good evidence for a beneficial effect of large dose vitamin C supplementation for chronic oxidative stress. The failure of vitamin E to reduce urinary excretion of 8-*epi*$PGF_{2\alpha}$ in smokers is difficult to reconcile with the beneficial effects of this vitamin in smokers on other indices of lipid peroxidation. Although speculative, it is possible that the relatively short supplementation period used in this study contributed to the lack of a significant effect.

Peroxidation of n-3 and n-6 PUFAs also leads to the production of breath ethane and pentane, respectively, which are volatile gases. Either in com-

Table 1. Antioxidant vitamins and biomarkers of lipid peroxidation

Source (first author)	Subjects	Design	Vitamin dose/day	Duration	Plasma vitamin level fold increase	Measured endpoint	Result
Conjugated dienes (CD), lipid hydroperoxides (LOOH), thiobarbituric acid-reactive substances (TBARS)							
Harats [9] 1990	17 smokers	measurements made before and after smoking 5–7 cigarettes over 90 min	study 1, n = 7 vitamin C 1,000 mg	2 weeks	2	plasma & LDL TBARS	A
			study 2, n = 10	4 weeks		plasma & LDL TBARS	
			n = 3 Control –		NC		NC
			n = 3 vitamin C 1,500 mg		2.3		A
			n = 4 vitamin E 600 mg		2.8		A
Brown [10] 1994	50 smokers	placebo-controlled 2 × 2 factorial, n = 25 per treatment	smokers vitamin E 280 mg	10 weeks	1.7	plasma TBARS, CD, and LOOH	A
	50 nonsmokers		nonsmokers vitamin E 280 mg		1.4		A
Cadenas [11] 1996	21 healthy men	placebo-controlled study, n = 7 per treatment	control –	30 days	ND	TBARS in urine	NC
			vitamin C 1,000 mg		ND		B
			vitamin E 100 mg		ND		B
					plasma / LDL		
Mol [12] 1997	14 nonsmokers	measurements made before and after supplementation period	vitamin E 600 IU	4 weeks	2.0 / 1.9	plasma TBARS	B
	12 smokers		vitamin E 600 IU	4 weeks	2.2 / 1.7		A
Wen [13] 1997	20 nonsmokers	measurements made before and after supplementation	n = 9 control –	4 weeks	NC	plasma TBARS	NC
			n = 11 vitamin C 1,000 mg		2.2		B
8-epi $PGF_{2\alpha}$							
Reilly [22] 1996	5 moderate smokers (15–30 cigarettes/day)	measurements made before and after supplementation	n = 5 moderate smokers vitamin E 100 IU	5 days	ND	Urinary 8-*epi*-$PGF_{2\alpha}$	B
	16 heavy smokers (> 30 cigarettes/day)		n = 7 heavy smokers vitamin E 800 IU	5 days	ND		B
			n = 5 heavy smokers vitamin C 2,000 mg	5 days	ND		A
			n = 4 heavy smokers vitamin C 2,000 mg and vitamin E 800 IU	5 days	ND		A

Table 1 (continued)

Source (first author)	Subjects	Design	Vitamin dose/day	Duration	Plasma vitamin level fold increase	Measured endpoint	Result
Breath pentane and ethane							
Hoshino [25] 1990	13 smokers	measurements made before and after supplementation	vitamin E 800 mg	2 weeks	2.6	breath pentane	A
Gottlieb [26] 1993	15 males	subjects were depleted in serum β-carotene by dietary manipulation then placed on high (n = 8) or low (n = 7) dose of β-carotene	β-carotene	4 weeks		breath pentane	
			high dose 120 mg		36 × baseline 79 × depletion		A
			low dose 15 mg		12 × baseline 36 × depletion		B
Allard [27] 1994	38 nonsmokers 25 smokers	randomized double-blind placebo-controlled trial	smokers	4 weeks		breath pentane/ethane	
			n = 11 placebo –		NC		NC
			n = 14 β-carotene 20 mg		11.7		B*
			nonsmokers	4 weeks		breath pentane/ethane	
			n = 20 placebo –		NC		NC
			n = 18 β-carotene 20 mg		8.5		B
Do [28] 1996	10 smokers 3 nonsmokers	measurements made before and after multivitamin supplementation	β-carotene 24 mg	3 weeks	11.3	breath ethane	C
			vitamin C 1,000 mg		ND		B
			vitamin E 800 IU		2.8		

NC = No change; ND = not done.
A = Significant ($p < 0.05$) vitamin protection (reduction in measured endpoint).
B = Not significant compared to placebo control (or baseline if no placebo group included).
C = Means were not different before and after treatment; however, significant effect if Wilcoxon sign rank test was used.
* Significant reduction in breath pentane output compared to baseline (week 0).

bination or individually, measurement of these expired gases in the breath of animals and man have generally been shown to increase with aging, cigarette smoking, vitamin E deficiency and acutely with exercise [23]. Thus, measurement of ethane or pentane in expired air has been suggested to offer a sensitive and noninvasive quantitative means to assess in vivo lipid peroxidation in human beings. Technical difficulties, particularly with the measurement of breath pentane, has limited the use of these indices of lipid peroxidation [23, 24].

The relationship between antioxidant vitamin status or intake and ethane or pentane levels in expired air has not been studied in great detail (table 1) [25–28]. As with other indices of lipid peroxidation, cigarette smokers have been used to examine this relationship. Hoshino et al. [25] supplemented 13 smokers with 800 mg/day of vitamin E for 2 weeks. Baseline levels of pentane were significantly higher in smokers ($p < 0.001$) than nonsmokers; supplementation with vitamin E significantly ($p < 0.001$) reduced these elevated pentane levels. Elevated ethane levels in the expired air of smokers have also been reported to be reduced with supplements of vitamin E (800 IU/day) in combination with vitamin C (1,000 mg/day) and β-carotene (24 mg/day) [28]. Of these three antioxidants, it is likely that only vitamins E and C were of benefit at the doses provided in this study, since a placebo-controlled trial by Allard et al. [27] failed to demonstrate that supplementation of smokers with β-carotene (20 mg/day) significantly reduced expired ethane levels. Thus supplementation of vitamin E and vitamin C may help to reduce lipid peroxidation in smokers, consistent with the above discussed studies using TBARS or F_2-isoprostanes as biomarkers of lipid oxidative damage. It should also be noted that in one study, β-carotene at relatively high doses (120 mg/day for 4 weeks) reduced pentane levels in expired air of normal subjects after a 2-week period of β-carotene depletion [26]. The importance of this observation remains to be determined.

Ex vivo LDL Oxidation as an Index of Oxidative Potential

Recent in vivo evidence implicates lipoprotein oxidation in the pathogenesis of atherosclerosis. Oxidized forms of LDL have been detected in atherosclerotic lesions from both animals [29, 30] and humans [31]. Moreover, lipophilic antioxidants have been shown to retard the development of atherosclerosis in hypercholesterolemic animals [32–34]. In vitro studies tend to support these in vivo observations since it has been demonstrated that oxidized LDL are chemotactic for monocytes [35], promote the ex vivo conversion of monocytes into lipid-laden foam cells [36, 37], and induce the production of cytokines and growth factors by cells of the vascular wall. The molecular mechanisms responsible for the in vivo oxidation of LDL are incompletely understood, however, considerable insight into this process has been obtained through the use of an in vitro assay [5]. In this assay freshly isolated LDL is incubated with a ROS source (e.g. transition metal ions such as Cu^{2+} or a peroxyl radical generator such as 2,2′-azobis-(2-amidinopropane)hydrochloride (AAPH) and the time course of LDL oxidation is monitored by measuring an index of lipid peroxidation, such as conjugated diene formation, lipid hydroperoxide formation or generation of TBARS. The kinetics of this process can then be used to quantify specific parameters such as lag phase (an index measure of the susceptibility of LDL to oxidation) or rate of diene conjugation (oxidation rate) during the propagation phase of lipid peroxidation (an index of the PUFA oxidizability in LDL) [5].

There have been a large number of studies examining the effects of specific antioxidant vitamins, either individually or in combination, on the ex vivo oxidation of LDL. Since we reviewed the small-scale clinical trials of LDL antioxidant protection up to 1993 [5], more information has become available on the influence of β-carotene and vitamins C and E on LDL lipid peroxidation (table 2) [38–51].

With a few exceptions, vitamin E has been shown to have a protective effect on the ex vivo oxidation of LDL in small clinical trials. In a recent placebo-controlled, randomized trial, Jialal et al. [41] examined the effect of vitamin E dose on the ex vivo oxidation of LDL. The diets of subjects (8 per group) were supplemented for 8 weeks with a placebo or one of the following doses of vitamin E: 60, 200, 400, 800 or 1,200 IU/day. Copper-mediated oxidation of LDL was assessed by monitoring the formation of conjugated dienes and TBARS. Vitamin E concentrations in plasma and LDL increased with all levels of vitamin E supplementation (e.g. % median LDL change at 8 weeks: 60 IU/day, 15 ± 4; 1,200 IU/day, 22 ± 12) and were not associated with changes in lipoprotein profile or in plasma concentrations of β-carotene or vitamin C. The minimum dose of vitamin E necessary to significantly decrease the susceptibility of LDL to oxidation (i.e. prolong the lag phase and decrease the oxidation rate) was 400 IU/day. Both plasma and LDL vitamin E concentrations correlated significantly with the lag phase and inversely with the rate of oxidation. In a similar placebo-controlled trial, Simons et al. [43] supplemented the diets of subjects (9–11 per group) with either placebo or one of following doses of vitamin E: 500, 1,000 or 1,500 IU daily. Consistent with the study of Jialal et al. [41], the lag time to LDL oxidation was significantly increased and the oxidation rate significantly slowed with vitamin E supplementation of 500 IU/day and greater. It is important to note that both the study of Jialal and the study of Simons were placebo-controlled trials and

Table 2. Antioxidant vitamins and ex vivo LDL lipid peroxidation (selected small trials since 1993)

Study (first author)	Subjects	Dose/day	Duration	Fold increase in plasma levels	Fold increase in LDL levels	Increase in LDL oxidation lag time	Decrease in propagation rate of LDL lipid peroxidation
Vitamin E							
McDowell [38]	16 patients with	placebo (n = 8)	8 weeks	NC	ND	–	–
1994	type IIa hyperlipidemia	800 IU (n = 8)		1.4	ND	NS ($p < 0.05$)*	ND
Suzukawa [39] 1995	8	150 IU for 1 week followed by 300 IU for 3 weeks	4 weeks	ND	1.9	$p < 0.01$	$p < 0.05$
Mol [40]	14 nonsmokers	600 IU	4 weeks	2	2	$p < 0.001$	$p < 0.01$
1997	12 smokers	600 IU	4 weeks	2	1.7	$p < 0.01$	NS
Jialal [41]	8	placebo	8 weeks	NC	NC	–	–
1995	8	60 IU	8 weeks	1.6	1.6	ND (NS)*	ND (NS)*
	8	200 IU	8 weeks	1.8	1.9	ND (NS)*	ND (NS)*
	8	400 IU	8 weeks	2.3	1.8	ND ($p < 0.05$)*	ND ($p < 0.01$)*
	8	800 IU	8 weeks	2.5	2.6	ND ($p < 0.05$)*	ND ($p < 0.01$)*
	8	1,200 IU	8 weeks	3.5	2.8	ND ($p < 0.001$)*	ND ($p < 0.01$)*
Princen [42]	20	no supplement (control)	consecutive	baseline	baseline	–	–
1995		25 IU	2-week	1.2	1.2	$p < 0.05$	NS
		50 IU	periods	1.2	1.3	$p < 0.05$	NS
		100 IU	with	1.4	1.4	$p < 0.05$	NS
		200 IU	increasing	1.7	1.5	$p < 0.05$	NS
		400 IU	dose	2.2	1.8	$p < 0.05$	$p < 0.05$
		800 IU		2.6	2.2	$p < 0.05$	$p < 0.05$
Simons [43]	11	placebo	6 weeks	1.1	1.2	–	–
1996	11	500 IU	6 weeks	2.0	1.8	ND ($p < 0.01$)*	ND ($p < 0.01$)*
	9	1,000 IU	6 weeks	2.1	1.9	ND ($p < 0.01$)*	ND ($p < 0.05$)*
	11	1,500 IU	6 weeks	2.5	2.0	ND ($p < 0.01$)*	ND ($p < 0.01$)*

Table 2 (continued)

Study (first author)	Subjects	Dose/day	Duration	Fold increase in plasma levels	Fold increase in LDL levels	Increase in LDL oxidation lag time	Decrease in propagation rate of LDL lipid peroxidation
β-Carotene							
Reaven [44]	6	placebo	6 weeks	NC	NC	–	–
1994	6	15 mg followed	4 weeks	9.5	9.5	NS	NS
		by 30 mg	2 weeks	11	11	NS	NS
Gaziano [45] 1995	16	25–50 mg	30 days	5.5	8.5	NS	NS
Fuller [46]	9 smokers	placebo	4 weeks	NC	NA	–	–
1996	10 smokers	1,000 mg	4 weeks	3.9	NA	NS ($p<0.025$)*	NS ($p<0.005$)*
Wen [47]	9 controls	–	4 weeks	NC	NA	–	–
1997	11 nonsmokers	1,000 mg	4 weeks	2.2	NA	NS	ND
Vitamin combination studies							
Nyyssonen [48]	20 smokers	placebo	3 months	NC	ND	–	–
1994	20 smokers	400 mg vitamin C	3 months	1.5	NA	$p<0.001$ (VLDL & LDL)	$p<0.04$ (VLDL & LDL)
		200 mg vitamin E		1.7	ND		
		30 mg β-carotene		3.1	ND		
		100 μg selenium		1.2	NA		
Gilligan [49] 1994	19 hypercholesterolemic patients	1,000 mg vitamin C	1 month	ND	NA	$p<0.001$	$p<0.001$
		800 IU vitamin E		ND	ND		
		30 mg β-carotene		ND	ND		
Abbey [50] 1995	15 smokers	145 mg vitamin C (in orange juice)	3 weeks	1.6	NA	NS	NS
		16 mg β-carotene (in carrot juice)		2.6	ND		
Mosca [51] 1997	45 patients with cardiovascular disease	1) placebo	12 weeks	NC	ND	–	ND
		2) 500 mg vitamin C	12 weeks	1.5	NA	NS	ND
		400 IU vitamin E		2	ND		
		12 mg β-carotene		6	ND		
		3) 1,000 mg vitamin C	12 weeks	2	NA	$p<0.02$	ND
		800 IU vitamin E		3	ND		
		24 mg β-carotene		10	ND		

NA = Not applicable; NC = no change; ND = not done; NS = not significant ($p<0.05$).
* Compared to baseline instead of placebo.
– = Placebo (control) group used for comparisons with treatment groups.

both failed to report their data based on comparisons with the placebo group. Thus, their results are based on comparisons with baseline information and their studies cannot technically be called placebo-controlled trials. One additional study examined the effect of vitamin E dose on the susceptibility of LDL to copper-induced oxidation [42]. The design of this study differed from those discussed above in that each of the 20 subjects enrolled ingested consecutively, during 2-week periods, 25, 50, 100, 200, 400 and 800 IU/day. This experimental design allows the subjects to be their own controls. LDL vitamin E concentrations increased linearly with dose as did the resistance of LDL to oxidation. Even at the lowest dose of vitamin E, 25 IU/day, a significant increase in lag time was observed. This contrasts with the study of Jialal et al. in which a dose of 400 IU/day was required for a significant increase in lag time. Both studies, however, agree that significant decreases in the copper ion-induce oxidation rate of LDL requires supplementation of at least 400 IU/day. Since it is currently uncertain how the results from these ex vivo studies relate to the situation in vivo, it is premature to make dietary recommendations based on this limited information.

Of some importance in evaluating ex vivo LDL oxidation studies in relation to vitamin E is the recently reported observation by Stocker's group [52] (which has subsequently been confirmed by other laboratories), that LDL-associated vitamin E can act as a pro-oxidant in vitro, initiating and propagating lipid peroxidation. This has been determined experimentally to occur at low radical flux rates. It is thought that the pro-oxidant activity of vitamin E results when co-antioxidants such as ubiquinol-10 and vitamin C are not available to react with and quench the vitamin E radical [53]. Thus, in the co-antioxidant-depleted environment of isolated LDL, vitamin E, when exposed to low radical fluxes, can act as a PUFA pro-oxidant. The results of in vitro oxidation studies, therefore, depend on both the vitamin E content of LDL and the specific incubation conditions used, in particular, the rate of radical production and the presence of co-antioxidants.

Since it is thought that β-carotene can function as an antioxidant this provitamin has been examined as to its efficacy in delaying the ex vivo oxidation of LDL. Despite reports that the antioxidant activity of β-carotene is most apparent at moderate concentrations and at reduced partial pressures of oxygen, Reaven et al. [44] have demonstrated that LDL isolated from subjects receiving β-carotene supplements do not inhibit ex vivo LDL oxidation. This was true regardless of LDL β-carotene content (0.26–2.84 mol/mol) or the oxygen tension at which the study was performed. Gaziano et al. [45] also found that LDL β-carotene content (0.29–2.47 nmol/mg LDL protein) does not enhance the ex vivo resistance of LDL to copper-induced oxidation. These studies, at least in the context of ex vivo LDL oxidation, do not support a role for β-carotene in the protection of LDL from oxidation.

The effect of vitamin C on the ex vivo oxidation of LDL has been little studied. This is largely due to the fact that vitamin C is a water-soluble antioxidant, and as such is removed from LDL during isolation from plasma. Interestingly, there is a relatively recent placebo-controlled trial that examined the ex vivo oxidation of LDL isolated from the plasma of cigarette smokers supplemented with relatively large doses of vitamin C [46]. Smokers (>1 pack/day for 5 years) were placed on a low vitamin C diet (<30 mg/day) for 2 weeks before being randomized to receive either placebo (n=9) or 1,000 mg/day of vitamin C (n=10) for 4 weeks. Plasma concentrations of vitamin C increased 600% over the course of the study in the supplemented subjects, but remained unchanged in the placebo group. Compared to the placebo group, vitamin C-supplemented smokers did not show significant changes in ex vivo LDL oxidation compared to controls (i.e. prolongation of the lag phase and a decreased oxidation rate). Significant effects on lag time and oxidation rate were observed only when comparisons were made with baseline measurements of LDL oxidizability. In a more recent study, in which LDL lag time was compared in both supplemented (vitamin C 1,000 mg/day for 4 weeks) and unsupplemented cigarette smokers, Wen et al. [47] were unable to detect a significant protective effect of vitamin C. Thus, the ex vivo oxidation of LDL appears to be little affected by dietary supplementation of vitamin C, a result to be expected based on the lipophobicity of vitamin C.

Studies that have supplemented subjects with antioxidant vitamins in combination prior to examining the ex vivo oxidation of LDL tend to support the observations of studies using individual vitamins. Thus, studies that included vitamin E in the supplement generally reported significant protection of LDL [48, 49, 51]. The dose of vitamin E in the supplement providing protection in placebo-controlled studies was in one case higher (800 IU/day) [51] and one case lower (200 IU/day) [48] than the effective dose reported by Jialal et al. [41] (400 IU/day) for the supplementation of vitamin E alone. Whether this reflects differences in study protocols, particularly the in vitro LDL oxidation conditions, or effects of other constituents of the supplements is unknown. In one trial, only β-carotene (16 mg/day) and vitamin C (145 mg/day) were supplemented in the diets of smokers by including orange and carrot juice (i.e. vitamin E was not part of the supplementation protocol) [50]. Although plasma concentrations of β-carotene and vitamin C increased 2.6- and 1.6-fold, respectively, during the supplement period (3 weeks) compared to the control period, the lag time to LDL oxidation and the LDL oxidation rate were not affected. Postoxidation LDL, obtained during the supplementation period, was reported to have significantly lower MDA concentrations in this study. Considering the issues related to the determination of MDA, the importance of this observation is unknown.

Relatively little is known concerning the in vivo events leading to the initiation of LDL lipid peroxidation. Whatever the mechanism, it is likely that plasma better represents the milieu in which oxidation occurs than isolated LDL in a buffer system. Thus ex vivo lipoprotein peroxidation studies in plasma with specific endpoints such as quantifying specific classes of lipid hydroperoxides or a specific class of lipid peroxidation endproducts such as F_2-isoprostanes may provide valuable new insights in the future.

Markers of Oxidative Damage to Proteins

The demonstration that oxidatively modified proteins can accumulate during aging and in pathologies such as atherosclerosis and cataractogenesis has focused attention on the mechanisms and products of protein oxidation. With the exception of cysteine, protein amino acids are not as reactive as lipids possessing bis allylic hydrogens in methylene carbon groups [54], and not surprisingly there are more studies that have examined antioxidation in lipids than proteins. As with lipids, protein oxidation may involve propagating radicals (e.g. alkoxyl radical) and results in a variety of reactive species (e.g. protein hydroperoxides) and stable products. Markers of protein oxidation include protein carbonyl derivatives, oxidized amino acid side chains, protein fragments, and formation of advanced glycation endproducts [54, 55].

Of the various indices of protein oxidation, protein carbonyl formation is the best studied. In a variety of tissues and organisms it has been demonstrated that oxidative stress increases protein carbonyl concentrations [55]. In addition, protein carbonyls increase with aging and in diseases associated with aging and premature aging (e.g. Alzheimer's disease and progeria) [55]. Protein carbonyl derivatives are generated by the oxidative cleavage of the peptide main chain or by oxidation of the following amino acid side chains: arginine, lysine, proline and threonine [54, 55]. In addition, α, β unsaturated aldehydes (e.g. HNE) generated during lipid peroxidation can form Michael addition adducts with specific amino side chains (cysteine, histidine and lysine) of proteins producing carbonyl derivatives. Carbonyl groups may also be introduced into proteins by adduct formation between the ε-amino group of lysine and either dialdehyde products of lipid peroxidation (e.g. MDA) or reducing sugars and their oxidation products [54, 55]. Thus there are a variety of pathways through which protein carbonyls are formed, not all of which are dependent on the direct oxidative modification of the protein. In addition, it should be noted that protein carbonyl measurements detect an incompletely characterized range of products. Thus, measurement of protein carbonyls in complex biological materials may not be suitable if one wishes to examine the direct effect of ROS on protein [54]. However, since carbonyls are usually formed by oxidative mechanisms, it would appear that assessment of this protein modification is likely to provide a reasonable index of oxidative stress.

In spite of the fact that the oxidation products of some amino acid side chains have not been fully characterized, some stable modifications of amino acids in addition to protein carbonyls have been suggested as potential biomarkers of protein oxidative damage. Thus, among others, methionine sulfoxide, ortho- and meta-tyrosine, dityrosine and 3-chlorotyrosine have all been suggested as markers of ROS injury [54, 56–58]. Determination of oxidized amino acid side chains in a given protein is potentially a powerful tool, since it can provide very specific information concerning the ROS involved, which may in turn help with strategies for the prevention of this oxidative damage. An example of this sort of specific amino acid oxidation marker is 3-chlorotyrosine. The presence of this modified amino acid in a protein indicates that the protein has been subjected to the products of myeloperoxidase [56]. The use of specifically modified amino acid side chains as biomarkers for ROS damage appears promising, however, the expense and complexity of this analysis may limit its use.

Nonenzymatic reactions of reducing sugars (e.g. glucose) and their oxidation products with protein amino groups (Maillard reactions) are thought to play an important role in protein aging and in the pathologies associated with aging and diabetes [54, 55, 59]. Thus, the protein products of glycation and glycoxidation have been proposed as biomarkers of oxidative stress. The structural elucidation of some of these Maillard reaction products remains a problem since a variety of products are formed and some are unstable. A few advanced glycation endproducts (AGE) have been identified. These include carboxymethyl lysine and carboxyethyl lysine (CML and CEL) and dibasic crosslinks such as pentosidine and glyoxal-lysine dimers [59–62]. Interestingly, it has recently been demonstrated that amino groups present on phospholipids such as phosphatidylethanolamine can also contribute to the formation of AGE products (e.g. carboxymethyl ethanolamine; CME) [59], and that CML can be a product of lipid peroxidation as well as glycoxidation [63]. These recent observations indicate that AGE products are a general reflection of carbonyl-amine chemistry and not a reflection of carbonyl (carbohydrate or lipid) or amine (protein or lipid) source. With this in mind, CME, CML and pentosidine have all been shown to increase in human skin collagen with age [60, 61, 64]. Although measurement of these products may potentially prove useful as biomarkers of certain types of oxidative stress (or complications relative to diabetes) their measurement is technically difficult. Perhaps as more is learned about suitable specific AGE products, immunochemical methods can be developed to more readily allow researchers to quantitate these products in human tissues or urine.

There are no relevant recent in vivo studies that have examined markers of protein oxidation in relation to some form of oxidative stress (e.g. cigarette smoking) and antioxidant vitamin status or supplementation.

Markers of Oxidative Damage to DNA

In regard to cancer, probably the most important target for ROS is DNA. At the molecular level damage to DNA can take many forms ranging from specifically oxidized purines and pyrimidines (more than 20 such oxidative lesions have been identified) to gross DNA changes such as sister chromatid exchange and the formation of micronuclei [2, 65, 66]. Specific DNA oxidation products accumulate depending on the ROS involved, its rate of production, and the cell's ability to protect or repair its DNA from the oxidative insult. Estimation of oxidized DNA repair products in the blood or urine are thought to reflect the overall rate of DNA damage to the body, while estimates of oxidative damage in accessible cells (e.g. leukocytes, colonic endothelium and buccal cells) reflect the balance between damage and repair (steady state) in the tissue examined [2].

Among the most promising biomarkers of oxidative damage to DNA is 8-oxo-guanine (8-oxoGua). The C-8 hydroxylation of guanine is one of the more frequent DNA base modifications observed with oxidative stress [2]. This lesion can be generated either by direct oxidation of the base in DNA or by the incorporation of the oxidized nucleoside triphosphate into DNA during synthesis or repair [2]. Generation of 8-oxoGua in DNA is a mutagenic and potentially carcinogenic event since the oxidized base has altered hydrogen bonding or 'coding specificity' preferentially forming base pairs with adenine rather than cytosine. Transversion mutations (G⇒T) result following replication of the oxidatively modified DNA [2, 65].

Current methodologies used to measure the C-8 hydroxylation product of guanine, either as 8-oxoGua or the nucleoside (8-hydroxy-2′-deoxyguanosine; 8-oxodG) are technically challenging. The methods involve DNA isolation and digestion (for cells and tissues) or multiple solid phase extractions (for urine) before product separation and quantitation by either gas chromatography/mass spectroscopy (GC/MS) with selective ion monitoring or HPLC followed by UV or electrochemical detection [2]. These two analytical methods have frequently provided quite different absolute values for the C-8 hydroxylation product of guanine in similar tissues. The methodological problems associated with this observation have only recently been elucidated and involve sample oxidation during preparation for analysis [2, 67]. It is also important to note that there are conflicting opinions concerning the suitability of measuring the C-8 hydroxylation product of guanine as a biomarker of the overall rate of oxidative DNA damage [2, 68]. It appears that at least in some animals diet may contribute to the urinary excretion of these products. In addition, the repair pathway responsible for removal of the oxidized base in vivo is still being debated. Thus, it is unclear if either the base or nucleoside is the more appropriate urinary marker.

An alternative approach to the determination of oxidized DNA bases by GC/MS or HPLC makes use of repair enzymes (e.g. endonuclease III) to introduce strand breaks at sites where oxidized bases are present [69]. The strand breaks in DNA from single cells (e.g. lymphocytes) can then be estimated by electrophoretic techniques. DNA strand breaks are susceptible to extension when an electric field is applied, therefore, the intensity of fluorescently stained DNA in extensions ('comet tails') can be semiquantitatively assessed and used as an index of strand breakage. This method, although not quantitative, may prove to be a useful tool since it can be employed to examine individual cells.

The evidence in favor of a critical role of antioxidant vitamins in the prevention of cancer comes primarily from epidemiological studies [4]. Recent studies, in human beings using biomarkers of oxidative damage to DNA as an index of potential mutagenic or carcinogenic events, have in general provided very limited support to the epidemiological observations (table 3) [70–76]. In a recent randomized placebo-controlled trial, Prieme et al. [76] failed to observe an effect of 2 months of supplementation with vitamin E (100 mg twice a day), ascorbic acid (250 mg twice a day) or coenzyme Q (30 mg twice a day) on oxidative DNA damage in smokers. DNA damage was estimated by the urinary excretion of the nucleoside 8-oxodG. These results agree with earlier less well controlled studies in smokers and nonsmokers that attempted to relate the urinary excretion of 8-oxodG with intake and/or plasma concentrations of β-carotene and vitamins E and C [73–75]. In contrast, steady-state estimates of cellular DNA oxidation have generally supported a role for antioxidant vitamins in the protection of DNA from oxidation [70–72]. Duthie et al. [72] using a DNA strand break 'comet assay' that specifically detected the oxidation of DNA pyrimidines, found that supplementation of the diets of smokers and nonsmokers with vitamin C (100 mg/day), vitamin E (280 mg/day) and β-carotene (25 mg/day) significantly ($p < 0.002$) reduced base damage in lymphocyte DNA. Similarly, Fraga et al. [71] have shown in humans that dietary vitamin C protects sperm DNA against endogenous oxidative injury. These investigators depleted vitamin C in seminal plasma by 50% through dietary manipulation and observed a significant ($p < 0.01$) increase in oxidative

Table 3. Antioxidant vitamins and biomarkers of oxidative DNA damage

Study (first author)	Subjects	Vitamin dose	Duration	Change in plasma levels	Marker	Results (change in marker)
Cell measurements (steady-state damage)						
Fraga [70] 1991	10 males	vitamin C 5 mg/day (depletion) vitamin C 10–20 mg/day (marginal) vitamin C 60–250 mg/day (repletion)	32 days 28 days 28 days	vitamin C 50% ↓ in seminal plasma vitamin C levels remain ≥ 50% ↓ vitamin C levels return to baseline	sperm 8-oxodG	↑, $p<0.01$ ↑, $p<0.01$ ↓, $p<0.01$
Fraga [71] 1996	51 males (22 smokers)	–	–	vitamin E 32% ↓ in seminal plasma of smokers vitamin C 17% ↓ in seminal plasma of smokers	sperm 8-oxodG	↑ in smokers
Duthie [72] 1996	male smokers and nonsmokers	25 mg/day β-carotene 100 mg/day vitamin C 280 mg/day vitamin E	20 weeks	– – –	lymphocyte strand break 'comet assay'	↓ $p<0.002$
Urinary measurement (net rate of damage)						
Witt [73] 1992	11	10 mg/day β-carotene 1,000 mg/day vitamin C 533 mg/day vitamin E	1 month	5.8-fold ↑ 1.3-fold ↑ 1.8-fold ↑	8-oxoG	no effect
Loft [74] 1992	83	intake of vitamins A, C and E, diet record	–	–	8-oxodG	not correlated
Van Poppel [75] 1995	119 male smokers	20 mg/day β-carotene (n = 62) placebo (n = 57)	14 weeks	13.7-fold ↑	8-oxodG	no effect
Prieme [76] 1997	142 male smokers	1) 200 mg/day vitamin E plus 500 mg/day vitamin C (n = 20) 2) 200 mg/day vitamin E (n = 20) 3) 500 mg/day vitamin C (n = 21) 4) 500 mg/day slow release vitamin C (n = 21) 5) 90 mg/day coenzyme Q_{10} (n = 40) 6) placebo (n = 20)	60 days	not done	8-oxodG	no effect

damage to sperm DNA as assessed by measurement of 8-oxodG. A more recent study by Fraga et al. [71] examined oxidative damage to sperm DNA in relation to the vitamin E and C status of seminal fluid in smokers. Smokers in this study had significantly ($p<0.005$) elevated concentrations of 8-oxodG in sperm DNA compared to nonsmokers, suggestive of increased oxidative stress. Seminal fluid concentrations of vitamin C and E were reduced in smokers, however, only the vitamin E concentrations were reduced significantly.

It is noteworthy that all of the studies examining the whole body rate of oxidative DNA damage (i.e. urinary excretion of 8-oxodG) failed to detect a relationship between intake and/or plasma concentrations of antioxidant vitamins and DNA damage. In contrast, studies examining 'steady-state' (tissue) levels of DNA damage consistently showed a beneficial effect of antioxidant vitamins on oxidative DNA damage. Whether this is the result 8-oxodG being a poor marker for the rate of DNA damage (as suggested by some investigators) or that all of the dilutional issues related to assessment of a whole body rate make this a less sensitive index of oxidative DNA damage await additional study. In any event, it appears that at least in some tissues and under some forms of oxidative stress antioxidant vitamins may prove beneficial in protecting DNA from oxidative damage.

Conclusions

In vivo oxidative damage is likely to occur at only a few sites or tissues at any given time, and since products of oxidation are subject to detoxification and metabolism, suitable biomarkers of in vivo oxidative damage have proven difficult to identify and validate. As might be expected considering these problems, there are relatively few reliable markers of in vivo oxidative damage and there have been few studies using these markers to assess the effects of dietary supplementation of antioxidant vitamins on lipid, protein or DNA oxidation. From the data reviewed, it appears that at least in smokers, supplementing the diet with vitamins C and E may prove beneficial in preventing oxidative damage to lipids and DNA. There is insufficient evidence to conclude that antioxidant vitamin supplementation in nonsmokers is of benefit. The doses of vitamin C (1,000 mg/day) and E (280 mg/day) required to reduce most indices of lipid peroxidation in smokers were without exception much higher than the present RDA. Since most of these studies did not attempt to define an optimal dose for protection, it is likely that doses lower than those reported may also prove beneficial. Clearly, in humans there are many unresolved questions concerning the efficacy of antioxidant vitamins to prevent oxidative damage and by inference, disease. As better in vivo markers of oxidative stress are developed, validated and used, our knowledge concerning the dietary requirements necessary to achieve and maintain optimal antioxidant concentrations at the plasma and tissue level should improve.

Acknowledgments

The authors are indebted to Barbara McVicar for assistance in the preparation of the manuscript. Work in B.F.'s laboratory is supported by grants from the US National Institutes of Health (HL-49954 and HL-56170).

References

1 Halliwell B, Chirico S: Lipid peroxidation: Its mechanism, measurement, and significance. Am J Clin Nutr 1993;57:715S–725S.
2 Loft S, Poulsen HE: Cancer risk and oxidative DNA damage in man. J Mol Med 1996;74:297–312.
3 Stahl W, Sies H: Antioxidant defense: Vitamins E and C and carotenoids. Diabetes 1997;46:S14–S18.
4 Bowen PE, Mobarhan S: Evidence from cancer intervention and biomarker studies and the development of biochemical markers. Am J Clin Nutr 1995;62:1403S–1409S.
5 Keaney JF Jr, Frei B: Antioxidant protection of low-density lipoprotein and its role in the prevention of atherosclerotic vascular disease; in Frei B (ed): Natural Antioxidants in Human Health and Disease. New York, Academic Press, 1994, chapt 11, pp 303–351.
6 Esterbauer H, Ramos P: Chemistry and pathophysiology of oxidation of LDL. Rev Physiol Biochem Pharmacol 1995;127:31–64.
7 Esterbauer H: Estimation of peroxidative damage. A critical review. Pathol Biol 1996;44:25–28.
8 Janero DR: Malondialdehyde and thiobarbituric acid reactivity as diagnostic indices of lipid peroxidation and peroxidative tissue injury. Free Radic Biol Med 1990;9:515–540.
9 Harats D, Ben-Naim M, Dabach Y, Hollander G, Havivi E, Stein O, Stein Y: Effect of vitamin C and E supplementation on susceptibility of plasma lipoproteins to peroxidation induced by acute smoking. Atherosclerosis 1990;85:47–54.
10 Brown KM, Morrice PC, Duthie GG: Vitamin E supplementation suppresses indexes of lipid peroxidation and platelet counts in blood of smokers and nonsmokers but plasma lipoprotein concentrations remain unchanged. Am J Clin Nutr 1994;60:383–387.
11 Cadenas S, Rojas C, Méndez J, Herrero A, Barja G: Vitamin E decreases urine lipid peroxidation products in young healthy human volunteers under normal conditions. Pharmacol Toxicol 1996;79:247–253.
12 Mol MJTM, de Rijke YB, Demacker PNM, Stalenhoef AFH: Plasma levels of lipid and cholesterol oxidation products and cytokines in diabetes mellitus and cigarette smoking: Effects of vitamin E treatment. Atherosclerosis 1997;129:169–176.
13 Wen Y, Cooke T, Feely J: The effect of pharmacological supplementation with vitamin C on low-density lipoprotein oxidation. Br J Clin Pharmacol 1997;44:94–97.
14 O'Brien KD, Alpers CE, Hokanson JE, Wang S, Chait A: Oxidation-specific epitopes in human coronary atherosclerosis are not limited to oxidized low-density lipoprotein. Circulation 1996;94:1216–1225.
15 Morrow JD, Hill KE, Burk RF, Nammour TM, Badr KF, Roberts LJ II: A series of prostaglandin F_2-like compounds are produced in vivo in humans by a non-cyclooxygenase, free radical-catalyzed mechanism. Proc Natl Acad Sci USA 1990;87:9383–9387.
16 FitzGerald GA, Tigges J, Barry P, Lawson JA: Markers of platelet activation and oxidant stress in atherothrombotic disease. Thromb Haemost 1997;78:280–284.

17 Fukunaga M, Makita N, Roberts LJ II, Morrow JD, Takahashi K, Badr KF: Evidence for the existence of F_2-isoprostane receptors on rat vascular smooth muscle cells. Am J Physiol 1993;264: 1619–1624.
18 Wang Z, Ciabattoni G, Créminon C, Lawson J, FitzGerald GA, Patrono C, Maclouf J: Immunological characterization of urinary 8-epi-prostaglandin $F_{2\alpha}$ excretion in man. J Pharmacol Exp Ther 1995;275:94–100.
19 Delanty N, Reilly MP, Pratico D, Lawson JA, McCarthy JF, Wood AE, Ohnishi ST, FitzGerald DJ, FitzGerald GA: 8-Epi-PF$G_{2\alpha}$ generation during coronary reperfusion. A potential quantitative marker of oxidant stress in vivo. Circulation 1997;95:2492–2499.
20 Pratico D, Lawson JA, FitzGerald GA: Cyclooxygenase-dependent formation of the isoprostane, 8-epi-prostaglandin $F_{2\alpha}$. J Biol Chem 1995;270:9800–9808.
21 Patrignani P, Santini G, Panara MR, Sciulli MG, Greco A, Rotondo MT, di Giamberardino M, Maclouf J, Ciabattoni G, Patrono C: Induction of prostaglandin endoperoxide synthase-2 in human monocytes associated with cyclooxygenase-dependent F_2-isoprostane formation. Br J Pharmacol 1996;118:1285–1293.
22 Reilly M, Delanty N, Lawson JA, FitzGerald GA: Modulation of oxidant stress in vivo in chronic cigarette smokers. Circulation 1996;94:19–25.
23 Kneepkens CMF, Lepage G, Roy CC: The potential of the hydrocarbon breath test as a measure of lipid peroxidation. Free Radic Biol Med 1994;17:127–160.
24 Springfield JR, Levitt MD: Pitfalls in the use of breath pentane measurements to assess lipid peroxidation. J Lipid Res 1994;35:1497–1504.
25 Hoshino E, Shariff R, Van Gossum A, Allard JP, Pichard C, Kurian R, Jeejeebhoy KN: Vitamin E suppresses increased lipid peroxidation in cigarette smokers. J Parenter Enter Nutr 1990;14: 300–305.
26 Gottlieb K, Zarling EJ, Mobarhan S, Bowen P, Sugerman S: β-Carotene decreases markers of lipid peroxidation in healthy volunteers. Nutr Cancer 1993;19:207–212.
27 Allard JP, Royall D, Kurian R, Muggli R, Jeejeebhoy KN: Effects of β-carotene supplementation on lipid perioxidation in humans. Am J Clin Nutr 1994;59:884–890.
28 Do BKQ, Garewal HS, Clements NC Jr, Peng YM, Habib MP: Exhaled ethane and antioxidant vitamin supplements in active smokers. Chest 1996;100:159–164.
29 Haberland ME, Fong D, Cheng L: Malondialdehyde-altered protein occurs in atheroma of Watanabe heritable hyperlipidemic rabbits. Science 1988;241:215–218.
30 Daugherty A, Zweifel BS, Sobel BE, Schonfeld G: Isolation of low density lipoprotein from atherosclerotic vascular tissue of Watanabe heritable hyperlipidemic rabbits. Arteriosclerosis 1988;8: 768–777.
31 Ylä-Herttuala S, Palinski W, Rosenfeld ME, Parthasarathy S, Carew TE, Butler S, Witztum JL, Steinberg D: Evidence for the presence of oxidatively modified low density lipoprotein in atherosclerotic lesions of rabbit and man. J Clin Invest 1989;84:1086–1095.
32 Kita T, Nagano Y, Yokode M, Ishii K, Kume N, Ooshima A, Yoshida H, Kawai C: Probucol prevents the progression of atherosclerosis in Watanabe heritable hyperlipidemic rabbit, an animal model for familial hypercholesterolemia. Proc Natl Acad Sci USA 1987;84:5928–5931.
33 Carew TE, Schwenke DC, Steinberg D: Antiatherogenic effect of probucol unrelated to its hypocholesterolemic effect: Evidence that antioxidants in vivo can selectively inhibit low density lipoprotein degradation in macrophage-rich fatty streaks and slow the progression of atherosclerosis in the Watanabe heritable hyperlipidemic rabbit. Proc Natl Acad Sci USA 1987;84:7725–7729.
34 Björkhem I, Henriksson-Freyschuss A, Breuer O, Diczfalusy U, Berglund L, Henriksson P: The antioxidant butylated hydroxytoluene protects against atherosclerosis. Arterioscler Thromb 1991; 11:15–22.
35 Quinn MT, Parthasarathy S, Fong LG, Steinberg D: Oxidatively modified low density lipoproteins: A potential role in recruitment and retention of monocyte/macrophages during atherogenesis. Proc Natl Acad Sci USA 1987;84:2995–2998.
36 Steinbrecher UP, Parthasarathy S, Leake DS, Witztum JL, Steinberg D: Modification of low density lipoprotein by endothelial cells involves lipid peroxidation and degradation of low density lipoprotein phospholipids. Proc Natl Acad Sci USA 1984;81:3883–3887.

37 Parthasarathy S, Steinbrecher UP, Barnett J, Witztum JL, Steinberg D: Essential role of phospholipase A_2 activity in endothelial cell-induced modification of low density lipoprotein. Proc Natl Acad Sci USA 1985;82:3000–3004.
38 McDowell IFW, Brennan GM, McEneny J, Young IS, Nicholls DP, McVeigh GE, Bruce I, Trimble ER, Johnston GD: The effect of probucol and vitamin E treatment on the oxidation of low-density lipoprotein and forearm vascular responses in humans. Eur J Clin Invest 1994;24:759–765.
39 Suzukawa M, Ishikawa T, Yoshida H, Nakamura H: Effect of in-vivo supplementation with low-dose vitamin E on susceptibility of low-density lipoprotein and high-density lipoprotein to oxidative modification. J Am Coll Nutr 1995;14:46–52.
40 Mol MJTM, de Rijke YB, Demacker PNM, Stalenhoef AFH: Plasma levels of lipid and cholesterol oxidation products and cytokines in diabetes mellitus and cigarette smoking: Effect of vitamin E treatment. Atherosclerosis 1997;129:169–176.
41 Jialal I, Fuller CJ, Huet BA: The effect of α-tocopherol supplementation on LDL oxidation. A dose-response study. Arterioscler Thromb Vasc Biol 1995;15:190–197.
42 Princen HMG, van Duyvenvoorde W, Buytenhek R, van der Laarse A, van Poppel G, Leuven JAG, van Hinsbergh VWM: Supplementation with low doses of vitamin E protects LDL from lipid peroxidation in men and women. Arterioscler Thromb Vasc Biol 1995;15:325–333.
43 Simons LA, Von Konigsmark M, Balasubramaniam S: What dose of vitamin E is required to reduce susceptibility of LDL to oxidation? Aust NZ J Med 1996;26:496–503.
44 Reaven PD, Ferguson E, Navab M, Powell FL: Susceptibility of human LDL to oxidative modification. Effects of variations in β-carotene concentration and oxygen tension. Arterioscler Thromb 1994;14:1162–1169.
45 Gaziano JM, Hatta A, Flynn M, Johnson EJ, Krinsky NI, Ridker PM, Hennekens CH, Frei B: Supplementation with β-carotene in vivo and in vitro does not inhibit low density lipoprotein oxidation. Atherosclerosis 1995;112:187–195.
46 Fuller CJ, Grundy SM, Norkus EP, Jialal I: Effect of ascorbate supplementation on low density lipoprotein oxidation in smokers. Atherosclerosis 1996;119:139–150.
47 Wen Y, Cooke T, Feely J: The effect of pharmacological supplementation with vitamin C on low-density lipoprotein oxidation. Br J Clin Pharmacol 1997;44:94–97.
48 Nyyssonen K, Porkkala E, Salonen R, Korpela H, Salonen JT: Increase in oxidation resistance of atherogenic serum lipoproteins following antioxidant supplementation: A randomized double-blind placebo-controlled clinical trial. Eur J Clin Nutr 1994;48:633–642.
49 Gilligan DM, Sack MN, Guetta V, Casino PR, Quyyumi AA, Rader DJ, Panza JA, Cannon RO III: Effect of antioxidant vitamins on low density lipoprotein oxidation and impaired endothelium-dependent vasodilation in patients with hypercholesterolemia. J Am Coll Cardiol 1994;24:1611–1617.
50 Abbey M, Noakes M, Nestel PJ: Dietary supplementation with orange and carot juice in cigarette smokers lowers oxidation products in copper-oxidized low-density lipoproteins. J Am Diet Assoc 1995;95:671–675.
51 Mosca L, Rubenfire M, Mandel C, Rock C, Tarshis T, Tsai A, Pearson T: Antioxidant nutrient supplementation reduces the susceptibility of low density lipoprotein to oxidation in patients with coronary artery disease. J Am Coll Cardiol 1997;30:392–399.
52 Bowry VW, Stocker R: Tocopherol-mediated peroxidation. The prooxidant effect of vitamin E on the radical-initiated oxidation of human low-density lipoprotein. J Am Chem Soc 1993;115:6029–6040.
53 Thomas SR, Neuzil J, Mohr D, Stocker R: Coantioxidants make α-tocopherol an efficient antoxidant for low-density lipoprotein. Am J Clin Nutr 1995;62:1357S–1364S.
54 Dean RT, Fu S, Stocker R, Davies MJ: Biochemistry and pathology of radical-mediated protein oxidation. Biochem J 1997;324:1–18.
55 Berlett BS, Stadtman ER: Protein oxidation in aging, disease, and oxidative stress. J Biol Chem 1997;272:20313–20316.
56 Hazen SL, Crowley JR, Mueller DM, Heinecke JW: Mass spectrometric quantification of 3-chlorotyrosine in human tissues with attomole sensitivity: A sensitive and specific marker for myeloperoxidase-catalyzed chlorination at sites of inflammation. Free Radic Biol Med 1997;23:909–916.

57 Huggins TG, Wells-Knecht MC, Detorie NA, Baynes JW, Thorpe SR: Formation of *o*-tyrosine and dityrosine in proteins during radiolytic and metal-catalyzed oxidation. J Biol Chem 1993;268: 12341–12347.
58 Wells-Knecht MC, Lyons TJ, McCance DR, Thorpe SR, Baynes JW: Age-dependent increase in *ortho*-tyrosine and methionine sulfoxide in human skin collagen is not accelerated in diabetes. Evidence against a generalized increase in oxidative stress in diabetes. J Clin Invest 1997;100:839–846.
59 Vlassara H: Recent progress in advanced glycation end products and diabetic complications. Diabetes 1997;46:S19–S25.
60 Sell DR, Monnier VM: Structure elucidation of a senescence cross-link from human extracellular matrix. Implication of pentoses in the aging process. J Biol Chem 1989;264:21597–21602.
61 Ahmed MU, Brinkmann Frye E, Degenhardt TP, Thorpe SR, Baynes JW: N^{ε}-(Carboxyethyl)lysine, a product of the chemical modification of proteins by methylglyoxal, increases with age in human lens proteins. Biochem J 1997;324:565–570.
62 Nagaraj RH, Shipanova IN, Faust FM: Protein cross-linking by the Maillard reaction. J Biol Chem 1996;271:19338–19345.
63 Fu MX, Requena JR, Jenkins AJ, Lyons TJ, Baynes JW, Thorpe SR: The advanced glycation end product, N^{ε}-(carboxymethyl)lysine, is a product of both lipid peroxidation and glycoxidation reactions. J Biol Chem 1996;271:9982–9986.
64 Requena JR, Ahmed MU, Fountain AW, Degenhardt TP, Reddy S, Perez C, Lyons TJ, Jenkins AJ, Baynes JW, Thorpe SR: Carboxymethylethanolamine, a biomarker of phospholipid modification during the Maillard reaction in vivo. J Biol Chem 1997;272:17473–17479.
65 Lindahl T: Instability and decay of the primary structure of DNA. Nature 1993;362:709–715.
66 Gerster H: Intermediate cancer biomarkers and their use in beta-carotene studies in humans. Int J Vitam Nutr Res 1996;66:3–18.
67 Ravanat JL, Turesky RJ, Gremaud E, Trudel LJ, Stadler RH: Determination of 8-oxoguanine in DNA by gas chromatography-mass spectrometry and HPLC-electrochemical detection: Overestimation of the background level of the oxidized base by the gas chromatography-mass spectrometry assay. Chem Res Toxicol 1995;8:1039–1045.
68 Collins AR, Dusinska M, Gedik CM, Stetina R: Oxidative damage to DNA: Do we have a reliable biomarker? Environ Health Perspect 1996;104:465–469.
69 Singh NP, McCoy MT, Tice RR, Schneider EL: A simple technique for quantitation of low levels of DNA damage in individual cells. Exp Cell Res 1988;175:184–191.
70 Fraga CG, Motchnik PA, Shigenaga MK, Helbock HJ, Jacob RA, Ames BN: Ascorbic acid protects against endogenous oxidative DNA damage in human sperm. Proc Natl Acad Sci USA 1991;88: 11003–11006.
71 Fraga CG, Motchnik PA, Wyrobek AJ, Rempel DM, Ames BN: Smoking and low antioxidant levels increase oxidative damage to sperm DNA. Mut Res 1996;351:199–203.
72 Duthie SJ, Ma A, Ross MA, Collins AR: Antioxidant supplementation decreases oxidative DNA damage in human lymphocytes. Cancer Res 1996;56:1291–1295.
73 Witt EH, Reznick AZ, Viguie CA, Starke-Reed P, Packer L: Exercise, oxidative damage and effects of antioxidant manipulation. J Nutr 1992;122:766–773.
74 Loft S, Vistisen K, Ewertz M, Tjønneland A, Overvad K, Poulsen HE: Oxidative DNA damage estimated by 8-hydroxydeoxyguanosine excretion in humans: Influence of smoking, gender and body mass index. Carcinogenesis 1992;13:2241–2247.
75 Van Poppel G, Poulsen H, Loft S, Verhagen H: No influence of beta-carotene on oxidative DNA damage in male smokers. J Nat Cancer Inst 1995;87:310–311.
76 Priemé H, Loft S, Nyyssönen K, Salonen JT, Poulsen HE: No effect of supplementation with vitamin E, ascorbic acid, or coenzyme Q10 on oxidative DNA damage estimated by 8-oxo-7,8-dihydro-2′-deoxyguanosine excretion in smokers. Am J Clin Nutr 1997;65:503–507.

Prof. Balz Frei, Linus Pauling Institute, Oregon State University,
571 Weniger Hall, Corvallis, OR 97331-6512 (USA)
Tel. +1 541 737 5075, Fax +1 541 737 5077, E-Mail balz.frei@orst.edu

Walter P, Hornig D, Moser U (eds): Functions of Vitamins beyond Recommended Dietary Allowances. Bibl Nutr Dieta. Basel, Karger, 2001, No 55, pp 68–79

Synergistic Effects of Antioxidant Vitamins

T. George Truscott

Chemistry Department, Keele University, Keele, Staffs., UK

Carotenoids (present in many fresh fruits and vegetables), vitamin E (present in wheat germ oils) and vitamin C (found in many citrus fruits) are often regarded as our most important dietary antioxidants, but little is known of their possible interactions. The aim of this work is to discuss such interactions and to suggest how this may lead to synergistic protective effects and also how deleterious effects may also arise.

Major topics will be the interaction of reactive oxygen species (ROS) with carotenoids (the ROS include peroxy radicals [$RO_2^{\bullet}$], NO_x and other species such as singlet oxygen and the toxic peroxynitrite anion, $OONO^-$), the interaction of carotenoids with each other as well as the interactions of the carotenoids with vitamins E and C.

Of the 600 or so carotenoids found in nature, about 40 are regularly consumed by humans. Carotenoids are commonly found in yellow, orange and green fruit and vegetables and naturally occurring carotenoids are added to food to enhance colour. Amongst the carotenoids often used as colourants are β-carotene, lycopene, lutein, astaxanthin and canthaxanthin. Such carotenoids can act as antioxidants both by quenching singlet oxygen and by scavenging free radicals but under some conditions pro-oxidant reactions may arise. This study concerns the free radical interactions of carotenoids and using recent results based on pulsed radiation techniques, we suggest molecular mechanisms for: (1) synergistic antioxidant protection by carotenoids with vitamins E and C, and (2) the switch from antioxidant to pro-oxidant behaviour as a function of oxygen concentration.

All the short-lived species (e.g. free radicals) are generated in a specific manner which allows their concentration to be monitored in a time-resolved manner and hence their reactivity to be studied. The fast-reaction techniques used are laser flash photolysis and pulse radiolysis and these methods are fully described in the literature [1].

The order of topics to be discussed will be: (1) The interaction of carotenoids with singlet oxygen. (2) The interaction of carotenes with vitamins C and E. (3) Cell membrane results and their explanation in terms of the interaction of carotenes with vitamin C and E. (4) Carotene oxy-radical interactions and a possible mechanism for the switch from anti- to pro-oxidant effects of β-carotene.

Interaction of Carotenoids with Singlet Oxygen

A considerable amount of work has been carried out on the quenching of singlet molecular oxygen ($^1O_2$) by carotenoids and how this reaction protects against $^1O_2$-mediated photo-oxidation reactions. In biological systems, molecules such as porphyrins, chlorophylls and riboflavin can sensitize $^1O_2$ production and this can lead to deleterious effects including DNA damage and lipid peroxidation.

Electron exchange energy transfer quenching is the principal mechanism of carotenoid photoprotection against $^1O_2$, although chemical quenching also occurs leading to destruction of the carotenoid. Energy transfer produces the carotenoid triplet state (^{3}CAR) via electronic energy transfer:

$$^1O_2 + CAR \rightarrow {}^3O_2 + {}^3CAR$$

Once produced, ^{3}CAR can easily return to the ground state dissipating the energy as heat or it can be quenched physically via enhanced intersystem crossing by $^3O_2$. Thus, the carotenoid acts as a catalyst-deactivating $^1O_2$.

Many different carotenoids have been studied to investigate the influence of different structural characteristics (fig. 1) on the ability to quench $^1O_2$. (Most of the data has been obtained using a germanium photodiode to detect the near infra-red luminescence of $^1O_2$ at $\approx$1,270 nm.) Typical results [2, 3], using benzene as solvent, are given in table 1.

As the number of conjugated double bonds increases, the energies of the excited states (S_2, S_1, T_1) decrease and, as can be seen, this is reflected in the dependence of the $^1O_2$ quenching rate constant on carotenoid chain length.

Conn et al. [2] also studied the 9- and 15-*cis* forms of β-carotene and showed that they have slightly lower reactivities towards $^1O_2$ than that of all-*trans*-β-carotene even though time-resolved resonance Raman studies have shown that they share a common relaxed triplet state. Also, interestingly, the

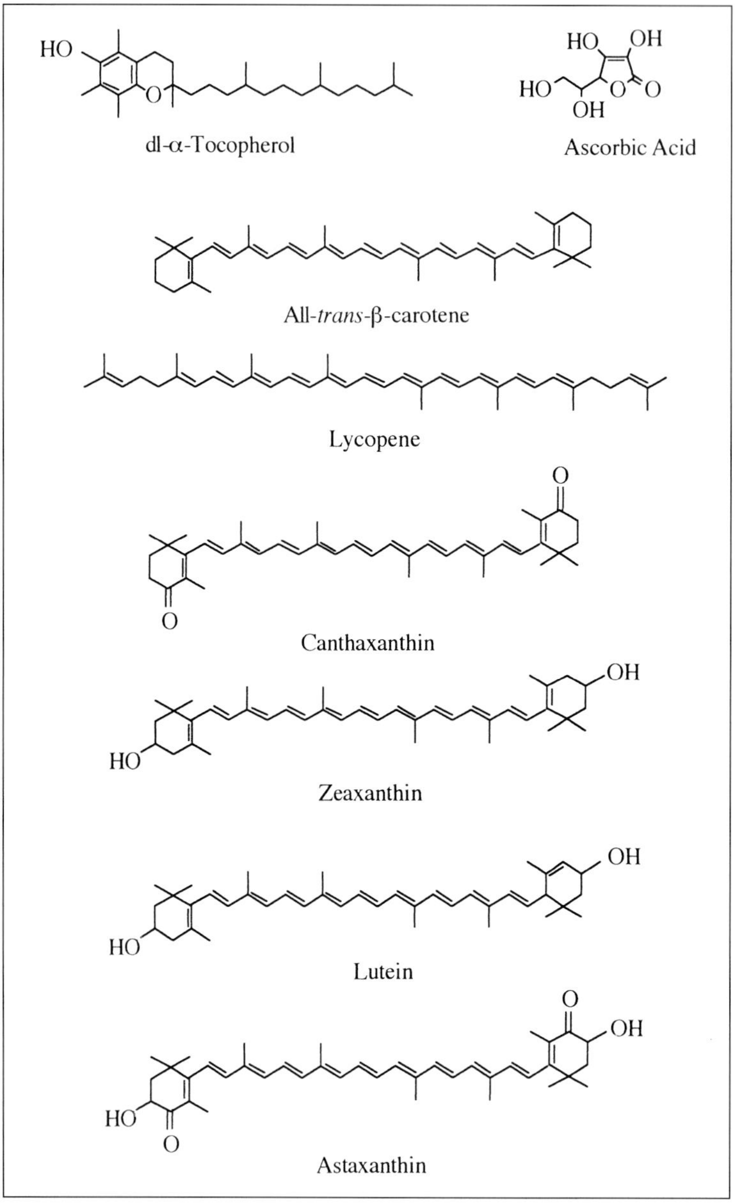

Fig. 1. Various carotenoids that have been studied to investigate the influence of different structural characteristics on the ability to quench $^1O_2$.

Table 1. Typical singlet oxygen quenching rate constants (k_q) for various carotenoids (with n conjugated double bonds) in benzene

Carotenoid	n	$k_q/10^9\ M^{-1}\ s^{-1}$
Dodecapreno-β-carotene	19	23.0
Decapreno-β-carotene	15	20.0
Tetradehydrolycopene	15	10.7
Astaxanthin	11 (+2, C=O)	14.0
Lycopene	11	17.0
all-*trans*-β-Carotene	11	13.0
15-*cis*-β-Carotene	11	11.0
9-*cis*-β-Carotene	11	11.0
Zeaxanthin	11	12.0
α-Carotene	10	12.0
β-apo-8-Carotenal	10	5.2
Lutein	10	6.64
Violaxanthin	9	16.0

two carotenoids in the eye, zeaxanthin and lutein, have very different quenching rate constants with respect to $^1O_2$. Zeaxanthin (n = 11) appears to be at least twice as effective as lutein (n = 10). Taken with a difference in radical reactivity (discussed below) this may indicate that they have different roles in the protection of the eye [3].

Di Mascio et al. [4] showed that lycopene is the naturally occurring carotenoid that quenches $^1O_2$ most efficiently, although their k_q value for lycopene is somewhat higher than that of other workers. However, although $k_q^{lycopene} > k_q^{\beta\text{-carotene}}$, this does not necessarily mean that it is a better antioxidant because lycopene is more susceptible to oxidation than β-carotene and may be used up more quickly (fig. 2).

Whilst showing that carotenoids are extremely good quenchers of $^1O_2$ in vitro, the studies so far discussed are not necessarily directly relevant to biological environments and little work has been carried out to test how effectively carotenoids protect cells against $^1O_2$-related damage.

Aqueous micellar solutions have been used as model biological environments. Haley and Truscott [5] studied $^1O_2$ quenching by carotenoids in 2% Triton X-100 and 4% mixed micelles (TX-405:TX-100, 3:1) in buffered pH 7 D_2O. There was no significant differences in the quenching rate constants for β-carotene in the two different micellar mediums ($k_q = 2.3 \times 10^9\ M^{-1}\ s^{-1}$ in TX-100 and $2.4 \times 10^9\ M^{-1}\ s^{-1}$ in mixed micelles). However, it is interesting to note that in the mixed micellar environment lycopene was no more effective

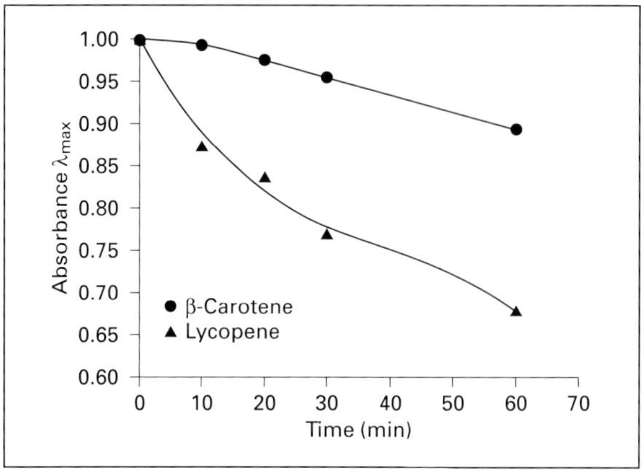

Fig. 2. Reduction in absorbance at λ_{max} of β-carotene and lycopene in hexane when bubbled with oxygen.

than β-carotene at quenching $^1O_2$ ($k_q = 2.0 \times 10^9$ M^{-1} s^{-1}), and therefore may offer no more protection against $^1O_2$ mediated damage in the physiological environment.

Anderson and Krinsky [6] studied the protective effect of β-carotene and canthaxanthin against damage to liposomes from dye-sensitized photo-oxidation. Incorporation of the carotenoids into the liposomal membrane gave good protection against the effects of the dye sensitization, with β-carotene offering the best protection. However, the carotenoids may not have been acting exclusively as $^1O_2$ quenchers, but also as radical quenchers. The same problem was found by Krinsky and Deneke [7] when they showed that β-carotene offered a protective effect in liposomes exposed to $^1O_2$ generated via decomposition of K_3CrO_8, which may have also generated superoxide and hydroxyl radicals.

Tinkler et al. [8] showed that four water-solubilized carotenoids bound to human lymphoid cells offered protection from dye-sensitized $^1O_2$. They used the technique of cell staining to determine how many cells had lethal membrane lesions, as well as monitoring the $^1O_2$ luminescence. The two techniques gave consistent results, with the highest protection being afforded by lycopene, followed by astaxanthin, β-carotene and canthaxanthin. The fact that lycopene is the most efficient C_{40} quencher agrees with the noncellular studies, but canthaxanthin showed better $^1O_2$ quenching than β-carotene in simple solvent systems, but in both of the more biologically relevant studies, it is a poorer quencher than β-carotene.

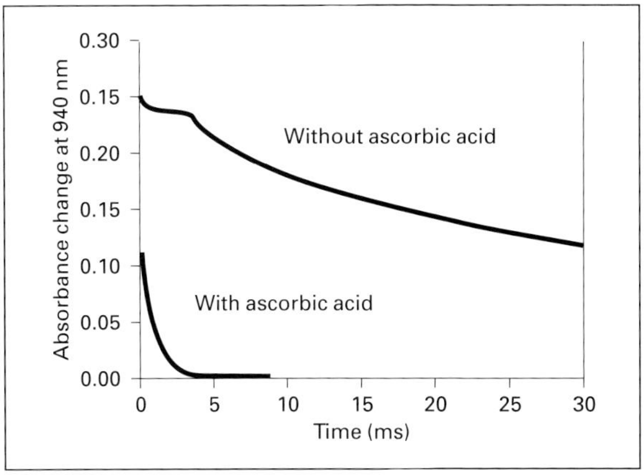

Fig. 3. Decay of β-$CAR^{\bullet +}$ following pulse radiolysis of 100 m*M* β-CAR in the absence and presence of 100 m*M* ascorbic acid in aqueous Triton X-100, pH 7.

Interaction of Carotenes with Vitamins C and E

Our investigations of the reactivity of ascorbic acid ($AscH_2$) with carotenoid radical cations, using pulse radiolysis and laser flash photolysis [9], have shown an enhanced $CAR^{\bullet +}$ decay rate in the presence of ascorbic acid (fig. 3), consistent with the following reactions in methanol (1) and water (2), Triton X-100 pH 7:

$$CAR^{\bullet +} + AscH_2 \rightarrow CAR + AscH^{\bullet} + H^+ \quad (1)$$

$$CAR^{\bullet +} + AscH^- \rightarrow CAR + AscH^{\bullet -} + H^+ \quad (2)$$

These reactions, for β-carotene, have second-order rate constants (±10%) of $9.4 \times 10^6\ M^{-1}\ s^{-1}$ in aqueous 2% Triton X-100 detergent micelles, pH 7, and $0.35 \times 10^9\ M^{-1}\ s^{-1}$ in methanol. The corresponding rate constants in methanol for the other carotenoids studied are given in table 2. Unfortunately, due to solubility problems, we could not obtain a value for lycopene.

We have also shown that in hexane several carotenoids (not astaxanthin) can repair vitamin E radical cation ($TOH^{\bullet +}$). We generate the radical cation of vitamin E ($TOH^{\bullet +}$) and observe the formation of $Car^{\bullet +}$ from the TOH radical. This we interpret as the reaction:

$$TOH^{\bullet +} + Car \rightarrow Car^{\bullet +} + TOH \quad (4)$$

Recently, for 7,7′-dihydro-β-carotene we monitored at wavelengths where $Car^{\bullet +}$ radicals absorb and at wavelengths where the $TOH^{\bullet +}$ radicals absorb and these

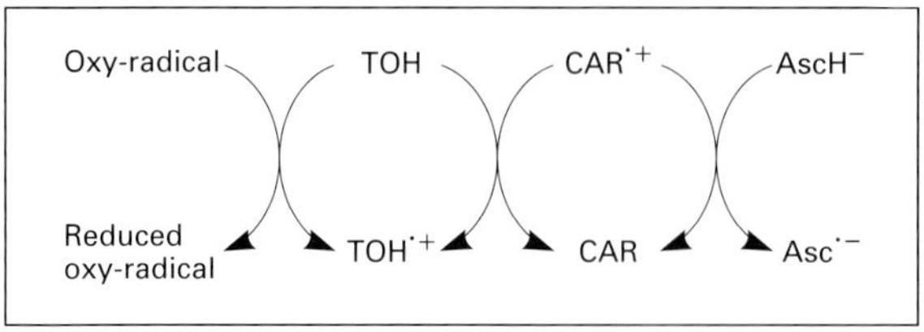

Fig. 4. Representation of oxidation-reduction processes.

Table 2. Second-order rate constants for the reactions of ascorbic acid and vitamin E with the carotenoids

Carotenoid	Rate constant for repair of $TOH^{\cdot+}$ by CAR $k/10^9\ M^{-1}\ s^{-1}$	Rate constant for repair of $CAR^{\cdot+}$ by $AscH^-$ $k/10^9\ M^{-1}\ s^{-1}$
Zeaxanthin	26.4	0.77
Mesozeaxanthin	23.3	0.82
7,7′-Dihydro-β-carotene	17.6	0.91
Lycopene	13.5	0.11
Septapreno-β-carotene	13.2	1.4
β-Carotene	10.2	0.35
Canthaxanthin	8.77	1.1
Lutein	5.31	1.3
β-apo-8-Carotenal	–	1.5

new results confirm that in nonpolar environments (hexane) the reaction we observe is:

$$TOH^{\cdot+} + CAR \rightarrow Car^{\cdot+} + TOH^{-} \quad (5)$$

However, in polar environments (alcohol) $TOH^{\cdot+}$ rapidly deprotonates to $TO^{\cdot}$ and we see no reaction between Car and $TO^{\cdot}$. The corresponding second-order rate constants for the reactions of both ascorbic acid and vitamin E with the carotenoids are given in table 2.

Overall, the scheme of oxidation-reduction processes which we observe can be represented as shown in figure 4.

A synergistic effect we have observed in cell protection by β-carotene and vitamins E and C (see below) may be related to the fact that β-carotene is not only quenching oxy-radicals but that the $CAR^{\cdot+}$ is re-converted to CAR. Of course, in hexane the β-carotene and α-tocopherol simply compete in scavenging any radicals present. However, a synergistic effect may reflect differing cellular locations of β-carotene and α-tocopherol. It is generally accepted that β-carotene is more lipophilic than α-tocopherol and will be more likely to be in the interior of a membrane. However, the β-carotene radical ($CAR^{\cdot +}$) is a charged species, while the α-tocopherol radical ($TO^{\cdot}$) is uncharged. Thus, the $CAR^{\cdot +}$ may re-orientate so that the charge is near the polar interface of the cell membrane and hence be more accessible to aqueous phase antioxidants such as ubiquitous ascorbic acid. Indeed, the discussion of Pryor et al. [10] also suggests the role of carotenoids as antioxidants depends on their environment. We are currently using time-resolved resonance Raman spectroscopy of carotenoid radical ions to investigate such effects.

The carotenoids associated with the eye (zeaxanthin and lutein) both contain terminal hydroxy groups and this may well mean that they are orientated so that these groups are near the polar interface, e.g. zeaxanthin may 'span' the membrane. The eye is subjected to a particularly harsh oxidizing environment and the protective role(s) of the carotenoids may be linked to the presence and orientation of these hydroxy derivatives. It was noted above that zeaxanthin was a more effective quencher of singlet oxygen than lutein and the radical quenching results show it is also a much more efficient quencher of $TOH^{\cdot +}$ than is lutein, possibly suggesting different roles in the protection of the eye for these carotenoids.

Cell Membrane Results and Their Explanation in Terms of the Interaction of Carotenes with Vitamins C and E

In collaboration with Dr. F. Böhm of the Charité Hospital, Berlin [see, e.g. 11, 12], we have investigated the ability of various antioxidant combinations to protect lymphocyte cells from destruction of the cell membrane by a range of oxidizing species. Typical results for the radical $NO_2^{\cdot}$ and the toxic peroxynitrite anion $OONO^-$ are listed in table 3.

As can be seen, there is a significant synergistic protection factor increase where all three antioxidants are present. In these experiments laser excitation at 355 nm is used to generate the oxy species. The $OONO^-$ anion is obtained by combination of the superoxide radical and NO, and, under the experimental conditions of this study, we cannot totally eliminate the generation of $NO_2^{\cdot}$. Nevertheless, $OONO^-$ is produced in these experiments and our data is at least consistent with carotenoid/vitamins E and C protection of cell membranes from this important in vivo oxidant.

Table 3. Membrane destruction of human lymphocytes, effect of antioxidants

Cells incubated with:	Reactive species	Percentage of stained cells	Protection factor
β-Carotene + vitamins E + C in vivo	$NO_2^{\cdot}$	6.0 (without 61.4)	10.2
β-Carotene in vivo	$NO_2^{\cdot}$	26.9 (without 53.2)	2.0
Vitamin E in vivo	$NO_2^{\cdot}$	7.6 (without 13.5)	1.8
Vitamin C in vivo	$NO_2^{\cdot}$	10.9 (without 13.5)	1.2
β-Carotene + vitamins E + C in vivo	$OONO^-$	5.2 (without 43.3)	8.4
β-Carotene in vivo	$OONO^-$	32.4 (without 55.1)	1.7
Vitamin E in vivo	$OONO^-$	7.7 (without 15.3)	2.0
Vitamin C in vivo	$OONO^-$	9.9 (without 13.7)	1.4

Carotene Oxy-Radical Interactions and a Possible Mechanism for the Switch from Anti- to Pro-Oxidant Effects of β-Carotene

The early work of Burton and Ingold [13] showed that at oxygen partial pressures up to 20% (i.e. atmospheric pressure) β-carotene inhibited the oxidation of two model compounds (methyl linoleate and tetralin) from peroxyl radicals produced via thermal decomposition of AIBN (azobisisobutyronitrile) in chlorobenzene. However, they showed that at higher oxygen partial pressures the initial rate of β-carotene autoxidation increases. Hence, it is a more efficient antioxidant at lower oxygen tensions. They also suggested that β-carotene may even become pro-oxidant at high oxygen partial pressures. Similar work by Jørgensen and Skibsted [14] in a heterogeneous lipid/water system, using metmyoglobin as the radical initiator, showed an antioxidant effect for four carotenoids, including β-carotene, even in 50% oxygen, although they still observed an increase in antioxidant efficiency with decreasing oxygen tension and several other studies, using heterogeneous environments such as microsomes and liposomes have shown the same effect.

Fast reaction techniques have also been used to study radical reactions with carotenoids in an attempt to gain a better understanding of their anti-/pro-oxidant effects. Thus, Hill et al. [15] showed that the $CCl_3O_2^{\bullet}$ radical reacted with carotenoids to yield an addition radical $(CCl_3O_2-CAR)^{\bullet}$ which subsequently formed the carotenoid radical cation $(CAR^{\bullet +})$:

$$CCl_3O_2^{\bullet} + CAR \rightarrow CCl_3O_2^{-} + CAR^{\bullet +}$$

$$\uparrow$$

$$CCl_3O_2^{\bullet} + CAR \rightarrow [CCl_3O_2-CAR]^{\bullet}$$

However, in the absence of oxygen, the carbon-centred radicals, e.g. $CCl_3^{\bullet}$, gave the radical cation via direct electron transfer. Also, carbon-centred radicals react efficiently with oxygen to give the corresponding peroxyl radical $(R^{\bullet} + O_2 \rightarrow RO_2^{\bullet})$ and this allows us to suggest schemes such as the following to explain a switch from anti- to pro-oxidant behaviour with increasing oxygen concentration:

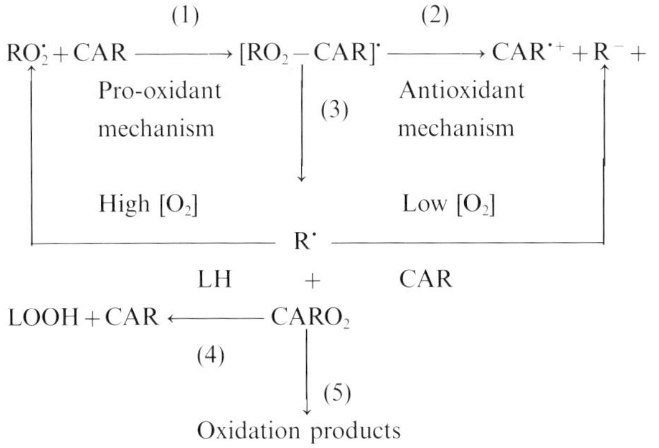

Of course, other steps can also be postulated such as:

$$(CAR - RO_2^{\bullet}) + O_2 \rightarrow {}^{\bullet}OO\text{-}CAR\text{-}RO_2$$

Our main speculation is that the key pro-oxidant step involves reactions such as the oxygen being 'carried' from a peroxyl radical to the lipid via the carotenoid and thus a dependency of the anti-pro-oxidation effect on oxygen concentration can arise. However, at the oxygen concentrations encountered in vivo, no pro-oxidant effect is to be expected.

Conclusions

(1) Of the retina carotenoids, zeaxanthin is more efficient than lutein at both quenching singlet oxygen and repairing vitamin E radical cation suggesting different protective roles in the macular for these carotenoids. (2) The radical cations of all the carotenoids studied were quenched by vitamin C and all carotenoids studied except, astaxanthin, repaired the radical cation of vitamin E. (3) Carotenoid radicals may lead to pro-oxidant deleterious effects if they are not removed by vitamin C; therefore, those with low levels of antioxidants, such as vitamin C (e.g. smokers) should probably supplement any carotenoids eaten with vitamin C. (4) The combination of carotene and vitamins C and E gave synergistic cell membrane protection. (5) Lycopene is the most readily oxidized carotenoid and astaxanthin radical cation is the most difficult to repair. The other carotenoids lie between these extremes and the biological significances of this scale of redox activity of carotenoids is worthy of future study.

Acknowledgements

Thanks are due to my collaborators: Drs Homer Black, Fritz Böhm, Ted Land, Louise Mulroy, Dave McGarvey, Tony Parker, Ms Ruth Edge and Ms Sue Tavender. Financial support is acknowledged from AICR EPSRC and The Wellcome Trust and F. Hoffmann-La Roche Ltd, Basel, Switzerland, are thanked for the supply of the carotenoids.

References

1 Bensasson RV, Land EJ, Truscott TG (eds): Excited States and Free Radicals in Biology and Medicine. Oxford, Oxford University Press, 1993.
2 Conn PF, Schalch W, Truscott TG: The singlet oxygen and carotenoid interaction. J Photochem Photobiol B 1991;11:41–47.
3 Edge R, McGarvey DJ, Truscott TG: The carotenoids as anti-oxidants – A review. J Photochem Photobiol B 1997;41:189–200.
4 Di Mascio P, Kaiser S, Sies H: Lycopene as the most efficient biological carotenoid singlet oxygen quencher. Arch Biochem Biophys 1989;274:532–538.
5 Haley J, Truscott TG: Unpublished results.
6 Anderson SM, Krinsky NI: Protective action of carotenoid pigments against photodynamic damage to liposomes. Photochem Photobiol 1973;18:403–408.
7 Krinsky NI, Deneke SM: The interaction of oxygen and oxy-radicals with carotenoids. J Nat Cancer Inst 1982;69:205–210.
8 Tinkler JH, Böhm F, Schalch W, Truscott TG: Dietary carotenoids protect human cells from damage. J Photochem Photobiol B 1994;26:283–285.
9 Böhm F, Edge R, Land EJ, McGarvey DJ, Truscott TG: Carotenoids enhance vitamin E antioxidant efficiency. J Am Chem Soc 1997;119:621–622.

10 Pryor WA, Cornicelli JA, Devall LJ, Tait B, Trivedi BK, Witiak DT, Wu MD: A rapid screening test to determine the antioxidant properties of natural and synthetic antioxidants. J Org Chem 1993;58:3521–3532.
11 Böhm F, Tinkler JH, Truscott TG: Carotenoids protect against cell membrane damage by the nitrogen dioxide radical. Nat Med 1995;1:98–99.
12 Böhm F, Edge R, McGarvey DJ, Truscott TG: β-Carotene with vitamins E and C offer synergistic cell protection against NO_x. FEBS Letters 1998;436:387–389.
13 Burton GW, Ingold KU: β-Carotene: An unusual type of lipid antioxidant. Science 1984;224: 569–573.
14 Jørgensen K, Skibsted LH: Carotenoid scavenging of radicals. Z Lebensm Unters Forsch 1993;196: 423–429.
15 Hill T, Land EJ, McGarvey DJ, Schalch W, Tinkler JH, Truscott TG: Interactions between carotenoids and the $CCl_3O_2^{\cdot}$ radical. J Am Chem Soc 1995;117:8322–8326.

Prof. T.G. Truscott, Department of Chemistry, Keele University, Keele, Staffs ST5 5BG (UK)
Tel. +44 1782 583038, Fax +44 1782 712378, E-Mail cha31@keele.ac.uk

Walter P, Hornig D, Moser U (eds): Functions of Vitamins beyond Recommended Dietary Allowances. Bibl Nutr Dieta. Basel, Karger, 2001, No 55, pp 80–91

Antioxidants and Chronic Disease: Evidence from Observational Epidemiology

Eric B. Rimm, Meir J. Stampfer

Departments of Epidemiology and Nutrition, Harvard School of Public Health, and Channing Laboratory, Department of Medicine, Brigham and Women's Hospital, Harvard Medical School, Boston, Mass., USA

Vitamin C, carotenoids and vitamin E, the three main dietary antioxidants, each affect lipid peroxidation and may reduce atherogenesis and lower risk of coronary heart disease (CHD). Antioxidants may also play a role in lowering risk of cancer, though most evidence from observational studies support a link for fruit and vegetable intake and not for any specific antioxidant. In this review we will focus on results from observational studies of antioxidant intake and risk of chronic disease.

Rapidly increasing evidence suggests that oxidation of low-density lipoprotein (LDL) is important in atherogenesis. As reviewed by Steinberg [1], oxidized LDL is preferentially taken up by macrophages to create foam cells. In addition, it appears to be cytotoxic to endothelial cells and decreases motility of tissue macrophages. Dietary antioxidants, including vitamin E and carotenoids such as α-carotene, β-carotene, and lycopene are fat-soluble and can function as free radical scavengers to decrease the initiation and propagation of fatty acid oxidation [2, 3]. In addition, vitamin E can inhibit smooth muscle cell proliferation and platelet adhesion [4], important components of atherogenesis. Although vitamin C is water-soluble and is not found in appreciable concentrations in LDL, it too has strong antioxidant capacity [5] and may function to regenerate or spare vitamin E [5, 6]. In addition to effects on atherosclerosis, antioxidants also may reduce free radical damage to DNA, a process believed to influence carcinogenesis. We review recent epidemiological findings which have addressed the role of these antioxidants in the prevention of chronic disease with a focus on cardiovascular disease.

Vitamin C

Although vitamin C is a strong antioxidant, the epidemiological evidence to support its role in lowering risk of cardiovascular disease is inconsistent. Results from cross-cultural studies suggest a strong inverse correlation between plasma levels of vitamin C and cardiovascular mortality [7]. These data are important in supporting the antioxidant hypothesis and for stimulating further research. However, other dietary and lifestyle characteristics also differ among the regions studied. One cannot definitively attribute the differences in cardiovascular disease specifically to dietary antioxidants; a multitude of other potential coronary risk factors must be considered. Moreover, it is unclear that within those countries, it is specifically the individuals with low levels of antioxidant intake who are at higher risk for disease.

Results from observational studies suggest that supplementary vitamin C intake to levels well above the US Recommended Dietary Allowance (RDA) (60 mg/day) does not lower risk of CHD. In a large prospective 4-year follow-up of 39,910 men in the Health Professionals Follow-Up Study, Rimm et al. [8] reported an age-adjusted relative risk (RR) of 0.83 for risk of CHD among men in the highest quintile (median intake 1,162 mg/day) compared to the lowest quintile (median intake 92 mg/day). However, after adjustment for intake of other antioxidants, such as carotenoids and vitamin E, the RR was substantially altered and was nonsignificantly positively associated with risk of CHD (RR1.25; 95% CI 0.91, 1.71). Among this population of health professionals, few men had intake levels below the RDA, thus the importance of vitamin C (diet or supplemental) in a population with a deficient dietary intake could not be evaluated. In a prospective study of 34,486 Iowa postmenopausal women [9], after 7 years of follow-up, the RR of death from CHD was 1.49 (95% CI 0.96, 2.30) between top and bottom quintiles of total vitamin C intake; the RR was similar when users of supplemental vitamin C were removed. As with the Health Professionals Follow-Up Study, even within the lowest quintile, intake of vitamin C among this population of women was well above the RDA. In a recent follow-up of 11,1178 persons from the Established Populations for Epidemiologic Studies of the Elderly (EPESE), vitamin C supplementaion alone had no effect on subsequent risk of coronary disease mortality [10]. Among participants reporting supplementation with vitamin C (and not vitamin E), the RR of CHD mortality was 1.00 (95% CI 0.74, 1.34). Recent evidence from an analysis of plasma vitamin C and risk of CHD in a cohort of 1,605 men from Finland provides some support for the hypothesis that very low levels of vitamin C intake may be associated with an elevated risk of CHD. Men with vitamin C deficiency had an RR of 3.5 (95% CI 1.8, 6.7) for subsequent myocardial infarction compared to men who were not deficient. Whether very low plasma levels of vitamin C or other dietary or lifestyle factors can explain this association is not well understood. Taken together, these results clearly exclude any appreciable cardiovascular benefit of vitamin C supplementation among populations with dietary intake at or above standard dietary guidelines.

To examine the direct role of vitamin C on atherogenesis, several studies have assessed atherosclerosis through carotid ultrasound or serial angiography. In a cross-sectional study of diet and carotid wall thickness, men and women > 55 years of age with lower intake of vitamin C had significantly higher average arterial wall thickness than those with the highest intake [11]. The association was somewhat attenuated after controlling for several nondietary factors. The overall inverse association for vitamin C among older men and women may be due to other diet or lifestyle characteristics associated with high dietary vitamin C intake in this study because little difference in wall thickness was reported between users and nonusers of vitamin C supplements. Furthermore, in a 2-year follow-up of 156 men with previous coronary artery bypass graft surgery, higher dietary or supplemental intake of vitamin C did not significantly alter the rate of coronary atherosclerosis as assessed by serial angiography [12].

In summary, the evidence for a cardioprotective effect of vitamin C is weak and inconsistent. Most observational studies find no benefit from higher dietary or supplemental intake of vitamin C. In several studies where dietary vitamin C reduces CHD, supplemental intake has little effect. This suggests that the association attributed to dietary vitamin C may be due to other diet or lifestyle factors among individuals with a high vitamin C diet. Although the importance of supplemental vitamin C among populations with deficient intake has not been thoroughly explored, there is little evidence to recommend vitamin C suplementation to reduce the risk of CHD.

The evidence linking vitamin C to lower risk of cancer is strongest for cancers of the lung [13] and stomach [14]. The details of specific studies are too numerous to mention in this review, but there is strong and consistent evidence from case-control and cohort studies that higher vitamin C status (either diet or serum) is associated with lower risk of lung and stomach cancer. Although biological mechanisms for a preventive role of vitamin C on cancer have been described, there is still the possibility that other components of vitamin C-containing fruits and vegetables are the responsible chemopreventive agents.

Carotenoids

Over the last several years, the epidemiological evidence to support the cardioprotective effect of carotenoids has grown, although the evidence supporting a specific benefit of β-carotene is inconsistent, and results from two large clinical trials suggest an adverse effect. Over 600 carotenoid compounds have been identified of which at least 40 have been isolated in foods; β-carotene, α-carotene, lycopene, β-cryptoxanthin, lutein and zeaxanthin are the most common [15]. Although the most recent results from clinical trials have focused on the health effects of only β-carotene, many previously published studies of cancer and cardiovascular disease have focused on other carotenoids as well.

In the 4-year follow-up of men from the Health Professionals Follow-Up Study [8], men consuming a diet high in total carotenoids had a significantly lower risk of developing CHD (supplemental β-carotene was only reported by 3% of the population and had little impact on the results). The strong inverse association was limited exclusively to men who were former or current smokers. These results were corroborated in a large European collaborative case-control study of adipose carotenoid concentrations and risk of nonfatal myocardial infarction [16] and a small nested case-control study in the US [17]. In both studies, the lower risk of CHD was limited to current or former smokers with high levels of carotenoids in adipose or serum. However, in the 13-year follow-up of the placebo arm of the Lipid Research Clinics Coronary Primary Prevention Trial (LRC-CPPT), a higher total serum carotenoid level was associated with a lower risk of subsequent CHD among current, former, and never smokers [11].

Several observational studies have reported strong inverse association between diets high in fruits and vegetables, specifically green leafy vegetables high in β-carotene, and risk of cancer [18] and heart disease [19]. From this and other supporting evidence, several long-term clinical trials were conducted to test the health effects of pharmacological doses of β-carotene. The clinical trials are reviewed in detail elsewhere in this publication, but consistent results from three large trials do not support the hypothesis that β-carotene supplementation of 20–30 mg/day is associated with lower risk of CHD [20–22]. Moreover, among men in the placebo arm of the ATBC study, baseline dietary and serum carotenoid levels also were not associated with a reduction in the incidence of angina [23]. Conersely, in a recent 8-year clinical trial of 1,188 men and 532 women designed to study β-carotene and nonmelanoma skin cancer, baseline plasma β-carotene concentrations were significantly inversely associated with cardiovascular disease deaths yet the B-carotene supplement (50 mg/day) did not decrease cardiovascular mortality [24].

Some have suggested that the apparent discrepancy in results between the clinical trials and observational studies may be due to chance or to insufficient follow-up time in some of the large trials. In fact, however, there is no discrepancy because no observational studies of β-carotene supplementation have been reported. Also, some have hypothesized that a β-carotene supplement among a population of long-term smokers (e.g. ATBC and CARET trials) may not be sufficient to counter the cardiovascular damage of oxidative stress caused by a lifetime of smoking. However, only 11% of men smoked in the Physicians Health Study and the β-carotene supplement was not beneficial to the smokers or nonsmokers. As discussed in detail elsewhere [15], β-carotene is only one of many carotenoids with strong antioxidant properties. Some [25], but not all studies [26], suggest that a daily regimen of β-carotene supplements may inhibit the absorption of other potentially important carotenoids. The inverse association between β-carotene and CHD from observational studies is most plausibly explained by other carotenoids or other dietary components found in fruits and vegetables with high β-carotene concentrations.

The epidemiologic evidence supporting the role of β-carotene in cancer prevention is based primarily on the large number of observational studies which have linked diets high in fruits and vegetables with lower rates of cancer [13, 14]. For lung cancer alone, results from 5 prospective and 18 case-control studies almost unanimously support the hypothesis that β-carotene or total carotenoids are inversely associated with risk of cancer [14]. Yet the evidence from clinical trials does not show that a β-carotene supplement lowers rates of lung cancer [20–22]. Although cancers of the bladder, breast, colon and other major sites have not been as strongly related to intake of carotenoids, evidence from observational studies does support an inverse association between lycopene and prostate cancer. Lycopene, a powerful antioxidant found in highest concentrations in tomato-based products, has been shown to be associated with lower risk of prostate cancer in a large prospective study of 47,894 US male health professionals [27]. Results from the Seventh Day Adventists Study [28] also support an inverse association between tomato intake and risk of prostate cancer. A better understanding of the physiologic consequences of a diet high in lycopene is needed.

In summary, the recent clinical trials convincingly demonstrate that β-carotene supplements do not lower the risk of CHD and cancer among men. More work is needed to determine if the cardiovascular and cancer benefit reported from the observational studies is attributable to other carotenoids or to other diet or lifestyle factors associated with a diet high in β-carotene.

Vitamin E

Vitamin E is predominantly carried in LDL and is particularly effective in protecting it from oxidation [3]. In addition, vitamin E can inhibit smooth muscle cell proliferation, an important component of atherogenesis [4]. Finally, vitamin E may reduce risk of cardiovascular disease through its effect on platelet adhesion [29]. Laboratory data and recent animal and epidemiologic data also support the hypothesis that vitamin E may reduce risk of cardiovascular disease [30]. In contrast, the observational studies of vitamin E and cancer are much less consistent and have focused on specific effects on cancer of the lung, cervix and colon [14].

In a cross-cultural study, Gey et al. [7] found a remarkable inverse correlation between plasma vitamin E levels (adjusted for cholesterol) and the rates of coronary mortality, even among the twelve centers with similar distributions of classical coronary risk factors. Similarly, Kristenson et al. [31] found lower plasma vitamin E in men from Vilnius (a high incidence region) compared to the lower risk area of Linköping, Sweden. In contrast, in the large EURAMIC case-control study of myocardial infarction from 10 centers in Europe, adipose tissue concentrations of α-tocopherol, assayed from 683 patients with acute myocardial infarction and 727 controls, were not associated with CHD risk. Indeed, those within the lowest quintile for α-tocopherol had a slightly (and nonsignificant) lower risk of myocardial infarction, with a multivariate odds ratio of 0.83 (95% CI, 0.57–1.21). In this European population it is likely that use of vitamin E supplements was very uncommon [16].

In a case-control study, Regnstrom et al. [32] found that LDL vitamin E levels were lower in cases than controls, and they observed an inverse relation between those levels and the coronary stenosis score.

Prospective designs are generally considered superior because the time sequence is clear; the exposure status is established before the diagnosis of disease. In a recent nested case-control study, Street et al. [17] assayed blood samples collected from adults in Washington County, Maryland. The individuals were all healthy at the time the blood was drawn. Vitamin E levels in serum from 123 participants who later developed myocardial infarction were compared with controls. For individuals in the lowest quintile for vitamin E (after adjustment for cholesterol), the RR was 1.4, but there was no consistent trend across the quintiles. In further analyses, Street et al. found a suggestion of a decreased risk of myocardial infarction among those with higher levels of serum α-tocopherol only in the group with higher levels of total cholesterol. However, that finding was not statistically significant.

In a larger study, Knekt et al. [33] ascertained dietary intake of vitamin E and other nutrients, in a cohort of 5,133 Finnish men and women aged 30–69, and followed them for 14 years for occurrence of new fatal CHD. When divided into tertiles of intake for vitamin E, the rates were lowest among men and women who consumed the highest amounts of vitamin E; trends were significant for both men and women. Only 3% of this population took supplements containing vitamin E or C. The analysis adjusted for age, smoking, serum cholesterol, hypertension, body-mass index and energy intake, but not other potential dietary and lifestyle confounders.

Meyer et al. [34] followed a cohort of 2,313 individuals, and found a significant reduction in the incidence of myocardial infarction among vitamin supplement users; the impact was most pronounced among users of vitamin E supplements.

In the largest study to date, Stampfer et al. [35] have reported results from the Nurses' Health Study. In this prospective cohort study, dietary data were collected in 1980 from 87,245 US female nurses aged 34–59, who were free from diagnosed cardiovascular disease and cancer at baseline. Participants were followed for 8 years using biennial questionnaires. During 679,485 person-years of follow-up, 437 nonfatal myocardial infarctions and 115 coronary deaths were documented. After adjustment for age and smoking, women in the highest fifth of the cohort for vitamin E consumption had an RR of 0.66 (95% CI 0.50–0.87). Further adjustment for other coronary risk factors and for dietary intake of other antioxidants had little impact. Virtually all of the effect was attributable to vitamin E from supplements, as all the women in the top 20% of vitamin E intake were users of either multivitamins or specific vitamin E supplements. Significant associations were observed only for intake of 100 IU/day or more; lower doses of vitamin E supplements had little effect. Women who used vitamin E supplements for less than 2 years had little apparent benefit, but use for 2 years or longer was associated with a 41% reduction in risk of CHD. These findings persisted after adjustment for intake of carotene and vitamin C, and use of multivitamins.

In the Health Professionals Follow-Up Study, Rimm et al. [8] prospectively studied 39,910 men aged 40–75 in 1986 and free of prevalent cardiovascular disease, diabetes or high cholesterol. During 139,883 person-years of follow-up, a total of 667 cases of fatal and nonfatal coronary disease were documented. Compared to men in the lowest fifth of vitamin E intake, men in the highest fifth had an age-adjusted RR of CHD of 0.59 (95% CI 0.47, 0.75). After adjustment for age, smoking, body size, caloric intake, dietary fiber intake, average alcohol consumption hypertension, aspirin use, physical activity, family history of heart disease profession, and intake of other antioxidant vitamins, the relative risks were essentially unchanged (RR 0.60; 95% CI, 0.44, 0.81). Smoking did not modify the associations for vitamin E.

In the Health Professionals Follow-Up Study, the contribution of vitamin E from foods and from supplements was examined separately. A significant reduction in risk of CHD was limited to those with intake of vitamin E from supplements, with only a modest inverse association between dose and CHD risk for doses of 100 IU/day or more. Compared to men who did not take vitamin E supplements, the maximal reduction in coronary risk was among men consuming 100–250 IU/day RR 0.54; 95% CI interval, 0.33, 0.88). The dose-response association for vitamin E from diet alone was suggestive of an inverse association (P_{trend} 0.11). However, limited variability in intake and error in measurement due to instability of vitamin E may have obscured a stronger association.

In another recent prospective study of antioxidants and CHD among women, Kushi et al. [9] reported a strong inverse association between dietary vitamin E (RR 0.38; 95% CI 0.18, 0.80 between extreme quintiles) and death from CHD in a subgroup limited to those who took no vitamin supplements. Overall, in the whole population, no significant trend was observed for dietary vitamin E. Unlike the Nurses' Health Study, participants who reported use of vitamin E supplements did not experience lower rates of CHD death during the 7 years of follow-up. Because no information was collected on duration of supplement use and only a small percentage of women reported taking at least 100 IU/day, results from this study cannot directly be compared with those from the Nurses' Health Study.

In another recent observational study of vitamin E intake and risk of CHD, Losonczy et al. [10] followed 11,178 elderly persons 67–105 years of age in the EPESE study. After an average of 8.5 years of follow-up a total of 1,101 coronary deaths were confirmed. Among participants reporting use of vitamin E supplements at baseline, the RR was 0.59 (95% CI 0.37, 0.93) for death from CHD compared to those not taking supplements. The risk reduction was not appreciably stronger among those taking both vitamin E and vitamin C supplements (RR 0.53, 95% CI 0.28, 0.97).

All of the above reviewed observational studies used clinically confirmed outcomes to evaluate risk reduction associated with vitamin E. However, exploring subclinical atherosclerosis progression provides valuable insight into underlying biological mechanisms. Hodis et al. [12] assessed the progression of coronary artery lesions using serial quantitative coronary angiographic methods among 162 nonsmoking men 40–59 years old. Subjects who took vitamin E supplements had significant reductions in lesion progression as compared to nonusers of supplements. The apparent benefit was limited to those taking 100 IU/day or more. In further follow-up from the same population, Azen et al. [36] reported a significant inverse association between vitamin E and early atherosclerosis as measured by high-resolution B-mode ultrasound of the distal common carotid artery. Similarly, in a cross-sectional survey of 1,187 asymptomatic participants in the EVA study, Bonithon-Kopp et al. [37] found that erythrocyte vitamin E was significantly and negatively associated with intima-media thickness of the common carotid artery in both men and women.

The observational studies suffer from the limitation that vitamin intake is self-selected by the study participants. Therefore, one cannot rule out the possibility that other characteristics of the health-conscious individuals who consume a healthy diet rich in antioxidant vitamins may also contribute to their reduced risk of developing CHD. To some extent, this potential confounding can be addressed if other coronary risk factors are ascertained. In the Nurses' and Health Professionals studies and the Iowa Women's Study, vitamin E supplement users did not differ markedly from nonusers in the prevalence of a wide array of risk factors, including diet [8, 9, 35]. Moreover, adjustment for these factors did not materially alter the risk estimates. However, one cannot adjust for unmeasured or unknown confounders. If the protective effect is due to some uknown factor, this factor would have to be very closely associated with vitamin E intake and a very powerful independent predictor of risk of CHD.

Further indirect evidence for a causal explanation from several of these studies is the finding that short-term use is not associated with benefit. Such a lag is consistent with the biology of the proposed mechanism, as vitamin E is thought to decrease atherosclerosis by reducing oxidation of LDL. In clinical trials of cholesterol-lowering to reduce atherosclerosis, it takes about 2 years of intervention before differences in clinical events begin to emerge. Thus, one would expect that an intervention operating through reduced atherosclerosis would take about 2 years before manifesting its benefit in terms of reduced clinical endpoints. Moreover, this 2-year lag which was observed for vitamin E also tends to refute the self-selection explanation, since self-selection pressures would operate most strongly at the time the self-selection began. Also, one would expect the same self-selection bias to operate for vitamin C supplements, but as discussed above vitamin C supplement users generally do not have lower risk. The most direct way to address this issue is through randomized trials, reviewed in detail elsewhere in this publication; evidence from the ATBC and CHAOS trials suggests that vitamin E supplementation may play a role in the primary and secondary prevention of CHD [20, 38].

The association (if any) for vitamin E and cancer appears to be much weaker [14] than for CHD and may only be limited to specific subpopulations [39]. Most of the evidence for vitamin E and lung cancer is derived from case-control studies with stored prediagnostic serum levels. Although 4 of 5 studies have found lower levels among cases than matched controls [40], evidence from prospective studies [14] and from the ATBC trial [41] do not support a strong effect.

Many observational studies have been conducted to examine the influence of vitamin E and cervical cancer. The evidence from the case-control studies is most consistent; OR between extreme tertiles or quartiles range from 0.4

to 0.7 [14]. However, the evidence from prospective observational studies is not as consistent [42, 43]. As with cardiovascular disease, the study of dietary vitamin E and cancer is difficult because the range of dietary vitamin E is limited. There are no published data on the association between vitamin E supplements and risk of cervical cancer.

In summary, results from observational studies support an effect of vitamin E supplementation on reducing risk of CHD with reasonable, though imperfect consistency. Evidence from the Nurses' Health Study [35], Health Professionals Follow-Up Study [8], CLAS study [12, 36], CHAOS study [38], and the Finnish ATBC trial [20, 23] suggest that the major effect, if any, is found at supplemental intake levels at or above 100 IU/day. If so, this could explain some of the inconsistent results for the effect of differences in plasma vitamin E levels on CHD risk in populations where supplementation is uncommon. The evidence for vitamin E and lower risk of cancer is less consistent. Some evidence suggests that high dietary intake of vitamin E may lower risk of cervical or lung cancer, but the associations are weak at best. In some studies of vitamin E from dietary sources, part or all of the apparent benefit could derive from other nutrients in the vitamin E-rich foods.

Because vitamin E has little toxicity [44, 45], the available evidence represents a promising approach to prevention of CHD, but not so for cancer. If the true magnitude of such an effect for cardiovascular disease is similar to that observed in the Health Professionals Follow-Up Study, the Nurses' Health Study, the EPESE study and the CHAOS study, then vitamin E supplementation could have a major impact on the incidence of CHD.

References

1 Steinberg D: Antioxidants and atherosclerosis. A current assessment. Circulation 1991;84:1420–1425.

2 Sies H, Stahl W: Vitamins E and C, β-carotene, and other carotenoids as antioxidants. Am J Clin Nutr 1995;62(suppl):1315S–1321S.

3 Princen HMG, van Poppel G, Vogelezang C, Buytenhek R, Kok FJ: Supplementation with vitamin E but not β-carotene in vivo protects low density lipoprotein from lipid peroxidation in vitro. Effect of cigarette smoking. Arterioscler Thromb 1992;12:554–562.

4 Boscoboinik D, Szewczyk A, Hensey C, Azzi A: Inhibition of cell proliferation by α-tocopherol: Role of protein kinase C. J Biol Chem 1991;266:6188–6194.

5 Retsky KL, Frei B: Vitamin C prevents metal ion-dependent initiation and propagation of lipid peroxidation in human low-density lipoprotein. Biochim Biophys Acta 1995;1257:279–287.

6 Jialal I, Grundy SM: Preservation of the endogenous antioxidants in low density lipoprotein by ascorbate but not probucol during oxidative modification. J Clin Invest 1991;87:597–601.

7 Gey KF, Moser UK, Jordan P, Stahelin HB, Eichholzer M, Ludin E: Increased risk of cardiovascular disease at suboptimal plasma concentrations of essential antioxidants: An epidemiological update with special attention to carotene and vitamin C. Am J Clin Nutr 1993;57(suppl):787S–797S.

8 Rimm EB, Stampfer MJ, Ascherio A, Giovannucci E, Colditz GA, Willett WC: Vitamin E consumption and the risk of coronary heart disease in men. N Engl J Med 1993;328:1450–1456.

9 Kushi LH, Folsom AR, Prineas RJ, Mink PJ, Wu Y, Bostick RM: Dietary antioxidant vitamins and death from coronary heart disease in postmenopausal women. N Engl J Med 1996;334:1156–1162.
10 Losonczy KG, Harris TB, Havlik RJ: Vitamin C supplement use and risk of all-cause and coronary heart disease mortality in older persons: The established populations for epidemiologic studies of the elderly. Am J Clin Nutr 1996;64:190–196.
11 Kritchevsky SB, Shimakawa T, Tell GS, Dennis B, Carpenter M, Eckfeldt JH, Peacher-Ryan H, Heiss G: Dietary antioxidants and carotid artery wall thickness – The ARIC Study. Circulation 1995;92:2142–2150.
12 Hodis HN, Mack WJ, LaBree L, Cashin-Hemphill L, Sevanian A, Johnson R, Azen SP: Serial coronary angiographic evidence that antioxidant vitamin intake reduces progression of coronary artery atherosclerosis. JAMA 1995;273:1849–1854.
13 Block G: Vitamin C and cancer prevention: The epidemiologic evidence. Am J Clin Nutr 1991; 53(suppl):270S–282S.
14 World Cancer Research Fund, American Institute for Cancer Research: Food, Nutrition and the Prevention of Cancer: A Global Perspective. Washington, American Institute for Cancer Research, 1997.
15 Krinsky NI: Actions of carotenoids in biological systems. Annu Rev Nutr 1993;13:561–587.
16 Kardinaal AF, Kok FJ, Ringstad J, Gomez-Aracena J, Mazaev VP, Kohlmeier L, Martin BC, Aro A, Kark JD, Delgado-Rodriguez M, et al: Antioxidants in adipose tissue and risk of myocardial infarction: The EURAMIC Study. Lancet 1993;342:1379–1384.
17 Street DA, Comstock GW, Salkeld RM, Schuep W, Klag MJ: Serum antioxidants and myocardial infarction. Are low levels of carotenoids and alpha-tocopherol risk factors for myocardial infarction? Circulation 1994;90:1154–1161.
18 Block G, Patterson B, Subar A: Fruit, vegetables, and cancer prevention: A review of the epidemiologic evidence. Nutr Cancer 1992;18:1–29.
19 Rimm E, Ascherio A, Giovannucci E, Stampfer M, Willett W: Dietary fiber intake and risk of coronary heart disease among a large population of US men (abstract). Am J Epidemiol 1995;141:S17.
20 The Alpha-Tocopherol Beta-Carotene Cancer Prevention Study Group: The effect of vitamin E and β-carotene on the incidence of lung cancer and other cancers in male smokers. N Engl J Med 1994;330:1029–1035.
21 Omenn GS, Goodman GE, Thornquist MD, Balmes J, Cullen MR, Glass A, Keogh JP, Meyskens FL, Valanis B, Williams JH, Barnhart S, Hammar S: Effects of a combination of β-carotene and vitamin A on lung cancer and cardiovascular disease. N Engl J Med 1996;334:1150–1155.
22 Hennekens CH, Buring JE, Manson JE, Stampfer MJ, Rosner B, Cook NR, Belanger C, LaMotte F, Gaziano JM, Ridker PM, Willett WC, Peto R: Lack of effect of long-term supplementation with β-carotene on the incidence of malignant neoplasms and cardiovascular disease. N Engl J Med 1996;334:1145–1149.
23 Rapola JM, Virtamo J, Haukka JK, Heinonen OP, Albanes D, Taylor PR, Huttunen JK: Effect of vitamin E and β-carotene on the incidence of angina pectoris – A randomized, double-blind, controlled trial. JAMA 1996;275:693–698.
24 Greenberg ER, Baron JA, Karagas MR, Stukel TA, Nierenberg DW, Stevens MM, Mandel JS, Haile RW: Mortality associated with low plasma concentration of β-carotene and the effect of oral supplementation. JAMA 1996;2275:699–703.
25 Kostic D, White WS, Olson JA: Intestinal absorption, serum clearance, and interactions between lutein and β-carotene when administered to human adults in separate or combined oral doses. Am J Clin Nutr 1995;62:604–610.
26 Ribaya-Mercado JD, Ordovas JM, Russel RM: Effect of β-carotene supplementation on the concentrations and distribution of carotenoids, vitamin E, vitamin A, and cholesterol in plasma lipoprotein and non-lipoprotein fractions in healthy older women. Am Coll Nutr 1995;14:614–620.
27 Giovannucci E, Ascherio A, Rimm EB, Stampfer MJ, Colditz GA, Willett WC: Intake of carotenoids and retinol in relation to risk of prostate cancer. J Natl Cancer Inst 1995;87:1767–1776.
28 Mills PK, Beeson WL, Phillips RL, Fraser GE: Cohort study of diet, lifestyle, and prostate cancer in Adventist men. Cancer 1989;64:598–604.

29 Steiner M: Vitamin E enhances the benefits of aspirin in preventing or reducting the incidence of strokes (abstract). Second International Congress on Antioxidant Vitamins and Beta-Carotene in Disease Prevention, Berlin, Oct 10–12, 1994, p 22.
30 Stampfer MJ, Rimm EB: Epidemiologic evidence for vitamin E in the prevention of cardiovascular disease. Am J Clin Nutr 1995;62(suppl):1365S–1369S.
31 Kristenson M, Zieden B, Kucinskiene Z, Schafer Elinder L, Bergdahl B, Elwing B, Abaravicius A, Razinkoviene L, Calkauskas H, Olsson AG: Antioxidant state and mortality from coronary heart disease in Lithuanian and Swedish men: Concomitant cross-sectional study of men aged 50. BMJ 1997;314:629–633.
32 Regnstrom J, Nilsson J, Moldeus P, Strom K, Bavenholm P, Tornvall P, Hamsten A: Inverse relation between the concentration of low-density-lipoprotein vitamin E and severity of coronary artery disease. Am J Clin Nutr 1996;63:377–385.
33 Knekt P, Reunanen A, Jarvinen R, Seppanen R, Heliovaara M, Aromaa A: Antioxidant vitamin intake and coronary mortality in a longitudinal population study. Am J Epidemiol 1994;139:1180–1189.
34 Meyer F, Bairati I, Dagenais GR: Lower ischemic heart disease incidence and mortality among vitamin supplement users. Can J Cardiol 1996;12:930–934.
35 Stampfer MJ, Hennekens CH, Manson JE, Colditz GA, Rosner B, Willett WC: Vitamin E consumption and the risk of coronary disease in women. N Engl J Med 1993;328:1444–1449.
36 Azen SP, Qian D, Mack WJ, Sevanian A, Selzer RH, Liu CR, Liu CH, Hodis HN: Effect of supplementary antioxidant vitamin intake on carotid arterial wall intima-media thickness in a controlled clinical trial of cholesterol lowering. Circulation 1996;94:2369–2372.
37 Bonithon-Kopp C, Coudray C, Berr C, Touboul P, Feve JM, Favier A, Ducimetiere P: Combined effects of lipid peroxidation and antioxidant status on carotid atherosclerosis in a population aged 59–71: The Eva Study. Am J Clin Nutr 1997;65:121–127.
38 Stephens NG, Parsons A, Schofield PM, Kelly F, Cheeseman K, Mitchinson MJ, Brown MJ: Randomised controlled trial of vitamin E in patients with coronary disease: Cambridge Heart Antioxidant Study (CHAOS). Lancet 1996;347:781–786.
39 Knekt P: Vitamin E and smoking and the risk of lung cancer. Ann NY Acad Sci 1993;686:280–287.
40 Knekt P: Vitamin E and cancer: Epidemiology. Ann NY Acad Sci 1992;669:269–279.
41 The Alpha-Tocopherol Beta-Carotene Cancer Prevention Study Group. The Alpha-Tocopherol, Beta-Carotene Lung Cancer Prevention Study: Design, methods, participant characteristics, and compliance. Ann Epidemiol 1994;4:1–10.
42 Batieha AM, Armenian HK, Norkus EP, Morris JS, Spate VE, Comstock GW: Serum micronutrients and the subsequent risk of cervical cancer in a population-based nested case-control study. Cancer Epidemiol Biomarkers Prev 1993;2:335–339.
43 Knekt P: Serum vitamin E level and risk of female cancers. Int J Epidemiol 1988;17:281–286.
44 Meydani SN, Meydani M, Rall LC, Morrow F, Blumber JB: Assessment of the safety of high-dose, short-term supplementation with vitamin E in healthy older adults. Am J Clin Nutr 1994;60:704-709.
45 Bendich A, Machlin L: Safety of oral intake of vitamin E. Am J Clin Nutr 1988;48:612–619.

Eric B. Rimm, Harvard School of Public Health, Department of Nutrition,
665 Huntington Avenue, Boston, MA 02115 (USA)
Tel. +1 617 1843, Fax +1 617 432 2435, E-Mail eric.rimm@channing.harvard.edu

Walter P, Hornig D, Moser U (eds): Functions of Vitamins beyond Recommended Dietary Allowances. Bibl Nutr Dieta. Basel, Karger, 2001, No 55, pp 92–134

Evidence from Intervention Studies

Hans K. Biesalski

Department of Biological Chemistry and Nutrition, University of Hohenheim, Stuttgart, Germany

An overwhelming amount of evidence from numerous epidemiological studies suggests that people who consume a diet rich in fruits and vegetables have a lower risk for several types of degenerative diseases.

From epidemiological data it was 'extracted' that increasing the plasma level of one of the 'markers' for vegetables (β-carotene) or fruit (vitamin C) intake should correlate with a decrease of a disease in a selected population. Since 1985, intervention studies with large populations were carried out with either β-carotene, vitamin E, vitamin C or varying combinations of these antioxidants. However, most of the studies failed to demonstrate the expected beneficial effect with respect to primary prevention. The question arises whether data from epidemiological studies can be taken as such for an interventional approach? Epidemiological studies usually show the result of a long-lasting dietary habit with respect to the development of a disease in a 'normal' population. This dietary habit is documented by usually one or in some cases more than one unproven biochemical marker for this dietary intake.

Accordingly, β-carotene stands for vegetables and some fruits, vitamin E for vegetable oils and vitamin C for fruits and vegetables. Intervention studies prove whether one or more of these 'markers' are the major preventive compound. However, fruits and vegetables contain a myriad of bioactive chemical components, both nutrient and nonnutrient by classification which beside β-carotene or vitamin E, alone or in combination might exert beneficial preventive effects.

Nevertheless, the supposition that β-carotene, vitamin E and vitamin C play a role in prevention of cancer, coronary heart disease (CHD), adult macular degeneration (ADM) and other diseases is based on experimental studies suggesting that these vitamins function as antioxidants, enhancers of immune function, modifiers of inflammatory processes and of signal transduction in and between cells. Thus, the totality of a great deal of epidemiological, animal, and in vitro evidence led to several intervention trials with different clinical endpoints mainly as cancer and some as CHD chemoprevention trials.

To answer the question whether there is any evidence from intervention studies for vitamin effects beyond RDA, the intervention studies are discussed based on their scientific rationale as recommended by Omenn (at the press conference during presentation of the Carotene and Retinol Efficacy Trial (CARET) Study. The scientific rationale for testing (chemopreventive) efficacy of (β-carotene, vitamin E, vitamin C) follows the outlined principals – epidemiology, presumed mechanism of action, in vitro model systems, animal models and human intermediate endpoints.

Lung Cancer

Epidemiology

More than 20 observational studies showed an inverse relationship between intake of vegetables (rich in carotenoids) and lung cancer in smokers [Van Poppel and Goldbohm, 1995]. Among all epidemiological cancer studies a vegetable-lung cancer relationship is predominant. Although these studies have contributed enormously to the literature regarding effects of carotenoids on cancer the interpretation of these studies is difficult for many reasons.

Fruits and vegetables are complex mixtures of vitamins, minerals, fibers, and numerous other phytochemicals. Thus, people who consume more carotenoids in their diet also consume more of these other substances, which might also be preventive. Also, individuals who consume more fruits and vegetables may also consume less dietary fat or may be more health conscious in other ways than individuals who consume relatively few fruits and vegetables. Observational epidemiological studies of carotenoids and human health must therefore be interpreted cautiously, as it is entirely possible that effects observed may result from dietary or other factors correlated with carotenoid intake rather than from carotenoids themselves.

The latter is of great importance if the blood level of one vitamin is taken as the major rationale for the preventive effect of a 'healthy diet'. The 'Basle Study' and others showed that people with high plasma β-carotene levels have a significant lower risk for lung cancer. Nomura et al. [1985] calculated a 7-fold risk increase in smokers with low plasma β-carotene levels (<0.2 μmol/l) as smokers with high levels (≥ 0.5 μmol/l). However, does this observation justify an intervention trial using β-carotene as a 'chemopreventive' drug?

Presumed Mechanism of Action

According to the *presumed mechanism of action*, β-carotene exerts preventive effects as a provitamin which is a source for retinoids and an efficient quencher of singulett oxygen. α- and β-Carotene slows growth of small cell lung cancer cells [Galligan et al., 1993]. However, due to the fact that it was not elucidated whether retinoids were formed, this growth-reducing effect cannot be solely attributed to α- or β-carotene. Retinoids are potent chemopreventive agents and their ability to control cellular growth and differentiation has been frequently documented. Even in established cancer cells retinoic acid can decrease neoplastic growth and induce normal differentiation [Jetten, 1991].

In vitro and Animal Models

From *in vitro studies* it can be concluded that vitamin A and its active metabolite retinoic acid are being involved in early lung cancerogenesis by controlling the normal appearance of the respiratory mucosa [Jetten et al., 1986] and avoiding the development of neoplastic transformation due to cigarette smoke condensate [Wolterbeek et al., 1995]. In addition, β-carotene quenches singulett oxygen and prevents lipid peroxidation at low oxygen tension. The ability of carotenoids to interfere with reactive oxygen species (ROS) and to prevent oxidative damage has been documented in numerous in vitro studies [Krinsky, 1993].

In laboratory studies, the carotenoids have antimutagenic and transformation inhibition properties in bacterial and cell culture systems. In Chinese hamster ovary cells, carotenoids block genotoxic damage by tumor promoters known to be oral carcinogens [Cozzi et al., 1997]. The precise mechanism of this prevention is unknown. Micronucleated cell frequency increases with genotoxic damage produced by carcinogens. β-Carotene, alone or with vitamin A, decreases micronucleated cell incidence in exfoliated human oral mucosal cells from high-risk populations [Stich et al., 1984; Weimann and Weiser, 1991].

The free radical mediated oxidation of benzo(a)pyrene, a procarcinogen occurring e.g. in cigarette smoke condensate, leads to the formation of an increased carcinogenicity [Kim et al., 1997]. β-Carotene might prevent the oxidation of benzo(a)pyrene and thereby it might reduce the risk for benzo(a)-pyrene-induced carcinogenesis. Indeed it was shown that dietary carotenoids reduce the enhanced carcinogenic potential of benzo(a)pyrene following free radical induced activation [Santamaria et al., 1983].

In addition, Edes et al. [1991] demonstrated that benzo(a)pyrene depletes vitamin A stores of different tissues and consequently promotes formation of squamous metaplasia. β-Carotene, however, prevents benzo(a)pyrene-induced vitamin A depletion. Vitamin A depletion of the respiratory mucosa favors the development of squamous metaplasia with a loss of ciliae and increase of mucus-secreting cells [Stofft et al., 1991] with the consequence of impaired mucociliary clearance. Loss of ciliae and hypersecretion (increase of goblet cells) is described in chronic obstructive pulmonary disease (COPD). COPD in smokers increases the risk for lung cancer [Demoly et al., 1994] and develops more frequently in people with lower vitamin A intake including B-carotene [Paiva et al., 1996].

Intermediate Endpoints

Whether COPD may serve as a *human intermediate endpoint* for lung cancer has to be further elucidated. Atypical cells in sputum might serve as premalignant endpoints for lung cancer. The Tyler (Texas) Chemoprevention Trial randomized 755 asbestos workers to receive β-carotene (50 mg/day) and retinol (25,000 IU every other day) vs. placebo to see whether the nutrient combination could reduce the prevalence of atypical cells in sputum. After a mean intervention period of 58 months, the prevalence of sputum atypia was nonsignificantly increased, not reduced, in the subjects receiving supplements [McLarty et al., 1995]. Supplemental β-carotene (20 mg/day), however, reduced micronuclei counts significantly in sputum from heavy smokers in a 14-week, randomized intervention trial [Princen et al., 1992]. The relevance of micronuclei to lung carcinogenesis is unknown. In studies dealing with cancer of the oral cavity however, micronuclei may serve as intermediate endpoints. With respect to the scientific knowledge about β-carotene discussed above, the justification to carry out intervention studies in smokers seems rather poor. In spite of good epidemiological evidence and accepted chemical action of β-carotene as 'inactivator' of carcinogenic ROS, the results from animal experiments are rather poor. Human intermediate endpoint studies with respect to lung cancer do not exist.

Intervention Studies

Two trials using lung cancer as a primary endpoint have now been completed. The α-Tocopherol β-Carotene (ATBC) Trial involved 29,133 males aged 50–69 years from Finland [The α-Tocopherol, β-Carotene Cancer Prevention Study Group, 1994] who were heavy cigarette smokers at entry (average 1 pack/day for 36 years). The study design was a two-by-two factorial with participants randomized to receive either supplemental α-tocopherol (50 mg/day), β-carotene (20 mg/day), the combination, or placebo for 5–8 years. Unexpectedly, participants receiving β-carotene (alone or in combination with vitamin E) had a significantly higher incidence of lung cancer (relative risk (RR) 1.18, 95% CI 1.03–1.36) and total mortality (RR 1.08, 95% CI 1.01–1.16) than participants receiving the placebo. Supplemental β-carotene did not affect

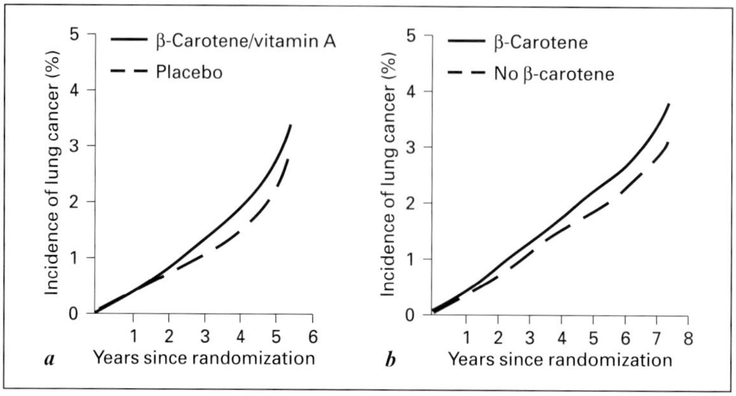

Fig. 1. Lung cancer incidence in CARET (***a***) and ATBC (***b***) study.

the incidence of other major cancers occurring in this population (prostate, bladder, colon/rectum, stomach). No data on COPD development or even existing COPD at start of the study are given. Within the placebo group, higher β-carotene intake from diet and serum β-carotene concentrations at baseline were associated with a lower subsequent lung cancer incidence (fig. 1).

Another surprising effect in the ATBC Study was the fact that the men who received doses of vitamin E (alone or with β-carotene) experienced 34% fewer cases of prostate cancer and 16% fewer cases of colon and rectal cancer than their peers, whereas their rates of lung cancer were unaffected. This finding has not been confirmed, however, and the ATBC Study was not designed to examine these correlations. The apparent decrease in prostate and colon and rectal cancers could either be a benefit of the vitamin E doses or just a chance occurrence. More trials are needed to explore this intriguing connection.

A second intervention trial (CARET) was recently published 2 years before the proposed termination [Omenn et al., 1996a]. CARET is a multicenter lung cancer prevention trial of supplemental β-carotene (30 mg/day) plus retinol (25,000 IU/day) vs. placebo in asbestos workers and smokers. Similar to the ATBC results, there was an RR of 1.36 (95% CI for weighted lung cancer incidence for the active intervention group compared with the placebo group, and RR 1.59 for weighted lung cancer mortality. All subgroups, except former smokers, had a point estimate of RR of 1.10 or greater for lung cancer. There are suggestions of associations of the excess lung cancer incidence with the highest quartile of alcohol intake (RR 1.99). CARET participants receiving the combination of β-carotene and vitamin A had no chemopreventive benefit and had excess lung cancer incidence and mortality.

With respect to the above discussed human intermediate endpoints, the presentation of subgroups data of the CARET study came out with interesting results [Chuwers et al., 1997]. The authors investigated the association between serum β-carotene or retinol concentration and level of ventilatory function in a population of asbestos-exposed men with a high rate of current and former cigarette smoking. The study population consisted of 816 subjects enrolled in the pilot component of the CARET. Serum β-carotene concentration was associated with FEV_1 ($p<0.05$) and FVC ($p<0.05$), with an approximately 100-ml increase over predicted values associated with raising the serum concentration from the 25th to the 75th percentile of the distribution in the study population (absolute difference 155 ng/ml), even after adjustment for the confounding effects of asbestos exposure and cigarette smoking. Raising the serum retinol concentration from the 25th to the 75th percentile (absolute difference 211 ng/ml) was associated with an approximately 70 ml increase in FVC ($p<0.05$) over the predicted value. These results provide support for the hypothesis that β-carotene and retinol may help to protect the respiratory mucosa against the deleterious effect of smoking and asbestos exposure and might help to prevent development of COPD. Indeed, low intake of vitamin A or low levels of plasma retinol are associated with a significant increased risk for COPD in smokers [Morabia et al., 1989, 1990].

In contrast to the findings from ATBC and CARET are results of an esophageal and gastric cancer prevention trial in China. The trial was conducted in residents from the general population of Linxian County. Nearly 30,000 men and women aged 40–69 took part in the study, which tested the efficacy of four different nutrient combinations at inhibiting the development of esophageal and gastric cancers. The nutrient combinations included retinol plus zinc, riboflavin plus niacin, ascorbic acid plus molybdenum, and the combination of β-carotene, selenium and α-tocopherol. After an intervention period of 5 years, those given the combination of β-carotene, vitamin E and selenium had a 13% reduction in cancer deaths (RR 0.87), a 9% reduction in total deaths (RR 0.91), a 4% reduction in esophageal cancer deaths (RR 0.96) and a 21% reduction in gastric cancer deaths (RR 0.79). None of the other nutrient combinations reduced gastric or esophageal cancer deaths significantly in this trial. This trial had limited statistical power for lung cancer with only 31 total lung cancer deaths [Blot et al., 1994]. However, the RR of death from lung cancer was 0.55 among those receiving the combination of β-carotene, α-tocopherol and selenium. The smoking prevalence, including individuals who had never smoked cigarettes for 6 or more months, was 30% in this study population. The study in China documented that a higher intake of vitamins (including β-carotene) might reduce cancer risk. However, it has to be considered that people living in this poor area were in a deficient state and have low vitamin plasma levels including retinol, β-carotene, vitamin E and C [Blot et al., 1993].

The fact that high plasma levels of either β-carotene or vitamin E indicate a far lower risk for cancer or cardiovascular diseases is well known. High plasma levels of these compounds however, are at least a result of a proper and consequently preventive nutrition. The evaluation of subgroups of the intervention studies give evidence that single vitamins such as vitamin E may have a benefit on prostate cancer incidence. Heinenen et al., [1998] described a 32% decrease in the incidence of prostate cancer among subjects receiving α-tocopherol (50 mg/day). Mortality was 41% lower in treated participants compared to controls.

Colon Cancer

Epidemiology

Cancers of the colon and rectum are a major cause of morbidity and mortality in most Western populations. There have been a number of epidemiological studies which suggest that dietary factors may play an important etiological role. However, there is some lack of agreement among various epidemiological studies as to the specific dietary risk and/or protective factors. Cases of colon and rectal cancer in many epidemiological studies reported a substantial excess intake of calories, protein, total fat, saturated fat, oleic acid and cholesterol when compared to both a neighborhood control series and a hospital-based control series. Although it is difficult to distinguish between the effects of these highly correlated nutrients, saturated fat generally yielded the highest and most significant RR estimates in most studies. Vegetable intake is clearly correlated with a reduced risk for colorectal cancer. Beside the high fiber content of vegetables, vitamins and carotenoids might play an important preventive role.

In Australia, Potter and McMichael [1986] found that vitamin C was protective for rectal cancer, whereas β-carotene and fiber intake were not associated with either colon or rectal cancer. Vegetables, as well as dietary and supplemental vitamin C, were associated with a significant protective effect for both colon and rectal cancer [Kune et al., 1987]. Fiber was protective only together with high vegetable intake. In a large study in Belgium [Tuyns, 1986; Tuyns et al., 1987], low consumption of raw vegetables conferred significant 2- to 3-fold excess risk. Green vegetables, tomatoes, and melon were significantly protective for both colon and rectal cancer, as was a carotenoid index, in Italy [La Vecchia et al., 1988]. In a study in Japan [Kato et al., 1990], daily raw vegetable consumption was significantly protective in rectal cancer, but weaker in colon cancer. In Hawaii [Heilbrun et al., 1989], rectal cancer cases had a nonsignificantly lower intake of green and yellow vegetables, fruits, cereals and legumes, as well as vitamin C and carotenoids. For colon cancer, there was an increased risk with low intake of vitamin C (RR 1.9, $p<0.01$), vegetables (except cruciferous) and fruit. Carotenoids were weaker and nonsignificant. Manousos et al. [1983] in Greece observed a significant protective effect for vegetables but not for grains, legumes or fruits.

In summary, for rectal cancer, significant relationships with fruit or vegetable intake were found in 7 out of 10 studies, with somewhat more support for fruit and vitamin C, and for raw vegetables rather than vegetables in general, and little support for cereal fiber. For colon as distinct from rectal cancer, most of the 25 studies were in the protective direction and 13 were significantly so. Most of the nonsignificant results were from older or smaller studies. At this site there is more support for vegetables and carotenoids, and in some studies cereal fiber has been found to be protective.

Taken together, there is some epidemiological evidence that carotenoids contribute to prevention of colorectal cancer. Very recently data from the nurses' health study were published [Giovannucci et al., 1998] which show a 75% lower risk for colon cancer in multivitamin users. This beneficial effect however was only evident after 15 years.

Presumed Mechanism of Action

The mechanism of action that may account for the cancer-inhibitory effect of β-carotene is not clearly understood but is presumed to be related directly or indirectly to its antioxidant activity. However, other effects, including inhibition of cellular proliferation and enhancement of the immune response, have also been attributed to β-carotene [Cahill and O'Morain, 1994; Murata et al., 1994]. At least the vitamin A activity of β-carotene may be responsible for the preventive effect. Indeed the antiproliferative effect of retinoids on colon cancer cells has been frequently documented [Kaleagasioglu et al., 1993; Kane et al., 1996].

ROS produce epithelial cellular injury. The detoxification of ROS and its cytotoxic metabolites is achieved by antioxidant enzymes [Hata et al., 1997] and through the presence of antioxidative vitamins. β-Carotene, which accumulates in human colonic neoplasmas and polyps [Maiani et al., 1995], inhibits proliferation of epithelial cells from normal human colonic mucosa [Frommel et al., 1995] and consequently may prevent polyp formation. From this it might be concluded that the concentration of β-carotene in the colonic mucosa is critically involved in early neoplastic transformation. This concentration might be regulated via the occurrence of fiber in the diet. A high-fiber diet may lead to a higher adsorption of carotenoids and other fat-soluble vitamins which will result in a higher concentration of these 'chemopreventive' compounds in the colonic lumen and at least the colonic mucosa. Indeed, animal models combining fiber and β-carotene have revealed a reduced formation of colonic aberrant crypts and tumor formation.

Animal Models

Alabaster et al. [1995] designed an experiment to evaluate the effects of β-carotene in the presence of high fat and low and high dietary level of wheat bran fiber using the Fischer-344 rat colon cancer model. Rats (20/group) were given either high fat (20% w/w), low wheat bran fiber (1% w/w) diets, or high fat (20% w/w) high wheat bran fiber (8% w/w) diets, with different levels of β-carotene. After 2 weeks of adaptation, half were given two weekly s.c. injections of azoxymethane (AOM, 15 mg/kg b.w.); and half two weekly s.c. injections of saline. Six weeks later, 5 rats from each dietary group were killed to evaluate the comparative effect of different dietary regimens on the induction of colon aberrant crypt foci (ACF). The remaining rats were maintained on their respective diets for an additional 20 weeks to examine the effect on colon tumor incidence. The total number of ACE/rat in the low-fiber groups declined from 44.0 ± 4.18 to 12.8 ± 1.95 in response to increasing amounts of β-carotene from 1 to 20 mg/kg diet. A similar progressive reduction in total ACE/rat was also seen in the high-fiber groups (20.8 ± 2.92 to 9.2 ± 0.50). ACF did not develop in the saline-exposed groups. Similarly, colon tumor incidence declined from 73 to 20% in high-fiber groups and from 27 to 13% in low-fiber groups in response to increasing amounts β-carotene from 1 to 20 mg/kg diet. The results showed that β-carotene and wheat bran, individually and when combined, protected the colon in rats consuming high-fat, Western-style diets from ACF and benign or malignant tumor formation.

In a second trial [Shivapurkar et al., 1995], the effect of dietary administration of a high-fat, low-fiber diet supplemented with vitamin E, β-carotene or folic acid and wheat bran on the growth of preexisting ACF that had been induced in Fischer-344 rats exposed to AOM and the diet for 10 weeks was evaluated. The rats were fed the diet for 2 weeks and were then given 2 s.c. injections of AOM while the rats continued on the diet. After 6 weeks, the rats were either maintained on the diet (control) or crossed over to a diet containing nontoxic levels of either vitamin E, β-carotene, folic acid or wheat bran. At 10, 14 and 18 weeks after the initiation of the experiment, the number of ACF with different multiplicities were compared between groups. The dietary intervention was continued for 30 weeks to determine whether the inhibitory effect on the growth of ACF influenced the subsequent development of colonic tumors. The results revealed that vitamin E and β-carotene caused a significant decrease in the number of ACF of different multiplicities when compared to the effect of the diet alone. The decrease in the number of ACF due to folic acid and wheat bran appeared to be much smaller and in most cases was not significant. However, there was also a significant decrease in the incidence of colonic tumors and tumor multiplicity in both the vitamin E and β-carotene groups that was not seen in the control group. The report clearly demonstrates the ability of vitamin E and β-carotene to inhibit the growth of colonic ACF, even in the presence of the strong promoting effect of high levels of dietary fat, using a postinitiation experimental design.

The results of these studies show that β-carotene might help to prevent colonic carcinogenesis on different steps (initiation, promotion). From several other experimental studies it can be concluded that β-carotene should be an effective chemopreventive agent against colon cancer formation.

Human Intermediate Endpoint Studies

Disappearance of polyps or biochemical markers for cancer formation, e.g. activity of the enzyme ornithine decarboxylase, were taken as 'intermediate endpoints'. A further biochemical marker for a higher risk might be the concentration of antioxidants in the colonic mucosa. Maiani et al. [1995] showed significant lower β-carotene levels in colon cancer and polyp patients compared to controls. In addition, they showed that β-carotene accumulates in human colonic polyps and cancerous tissue. The increase in β-carotene concentration after supplementation in cancerous lesions indicates that the relatively low initial levels were not related to an inability of the colon to accumulate β-carotene but is probably due to low consumption of foods containing β-carotene or at least rapid metabolism of β-carotene at the local or systemic level in these patients.

To determine whether patients with colon cancer metabolize β-carotene differently from benign colon polyp patients, a normal control group (n = 13) and groups of resected colon polyp patients (n = 29) or resected colon cancer patients were supplemented with placebo or β-carotene (30 mg/day) for 3 months [Tang et al., 1995]. Serum samples at zero and after 3 months of the study were analyzed for retinoic acid and β-carotene. The results showed that β-carotene levels in the serum of colon polyp and colon cancer groups were 8- to 12-fold higher than the untreated control or the placebo-treated groups. The benign polyp subjects (n = 17) receiving β-carotene showed a significant rise in serum *trans*-retinoic acid after 3 months. The *trans*-retinoic acid values from the colon cancer receiving β-carotene (n = 11) or placebo (n = 10) group were significantly lower than the values from the β-carotene-supplemented colon polyp group.

The data show that either metabolization or uptake of β-carotene is impaired in polyp and colon cancer patients. β-Carotene concentration and at least sufficient metabolism might control early steps of either polyp or cancer formation. At least the metabolite of β-carotene retinoic acid might help to control colonic cell proliferation as a critical step. However, it is not known if the rate of colonic cell proliferation differs among individuals with or without a history of colonic polyps or cancer and if proliferation changes in response to β-carotene. Frommel et al. [1995] tried to elucidate whether differences exist in colonic cell proliferation in individuals with and without prior colonic polyps or tumors and whether β-carotene accumulates in colonic mucosa following dietary supplementation, and whether mucosal β-carotene accumulation influences colonic cell proliferation. The participants included 20 individuals with normal colons (as judged by recent colonoscopy), 40 with a history of colonic polyp(s) and 41 with prior colon cancer.

Cellular proliferation was assessed on the basis of tissue ornithine decarboxylase (ODC) activity, urinary polyamine excretion, and proliferation cell nuclear antigen expression. Colonic cell proliferation did not differ in samples obtained from individuals with and without prior colonic polyp(s) or cancer, β-carotene concentrations in serum and colonic tissue were significantly increased in groups receiving β-carotene ($p < 0.001$). However, cell proliferation did not differ, as judged by any of the three measures, among samples from experimental groups collected before and after supplementation with β-carotene. In conclusion, dietary supplementation with β-carotene for a period of 3 months does not alter colonic cell proliferation in individuals with a history of colonic polyps or cancer.

In contrast it was shown that plasma β-carotene concentration following supplementation is inversely correlated with ODC expression in the rectal mucosa of colon cancer patients [Phillips et al., 1993]. 20 male subjects who had previously undergone resection of colonic adenocarcinoma were studied. Each subject received β-carotene, 30 mg orally, daily for 6 months. Rectal mucosa was sampled at multiple intervals prior to, during and following β-carotene administration. Mucosal ODC activity and serum and mucosal β-carotene concentrations were determined at each interval. ODC activity was inhibited by 44% ($p < 0.05$) and 57% ($p < 0.01$) after 2 and 9 weeks of β-carotene administration respectively, and remained low compared with baseline even 6 months following discontinuation of β-carotene. The authors suggest that the demonstrated inhibition of rectal mucosal ODC activity in these patients with resected colon cancer may prove β-carotene useful as a cancer-chemopreventive agent. The reduction of ODC might be a consequence of retinoic acid formation from β-carotene. Very recently we showed that retinoic acid efficiently reduces UVB-induced expression of ODC in human skin fibroblasts [Francz et al., 1998].

A decrease in ODC activity reflects a decrease in the rate of cell proliferation and is suggestive evidence of inhibition of the precancerous process. According to experimental data, the action of tumor promoters correlates with their ability to induce ODC activity in target tissues [O'Brien et al., 1975; Verma, 1990]. Moreover, in many experimental in vivo models, the suppression of ODC activity by irreversible inhibition of the enzyme α-difluoromethylornithine decreases tumor incidence [Janne and Alhonen-Hongleuro, 1998; Verma, 1990]. Therefore, it may be suggested that abnormally high levels of ODC activity may serve not only as a marker of carcinogenesis but may play an essential role in the biochemical mechanism of this stage of carcinogenesis. Higher levels of ODC might be a result of increased formation of ROS. For example, UVB irradiation induces formation of ROS and an increase of ODC expression. As a consequence antioxidative vitamins reduce oxidative stress and subsequently decrease ODC formation. At least it cannot be ruled out that the decrease in ODC activity is indirectly related with the well-known capacity of β-carotene to enhance gap junction communications [Zhang et al., 1991] that inhibit initiated cells from progressing to cells expressing the neoplastic phenotype. The latter may be linked with the conversion of β-carotene in target tissues to retinoic acid [Wang et al., 1992], which has a significant role in cell differentiation. It is possible that all mechanisms mentioned above may play a role in the downregulation of ODC expression.

Based on these data, β-carotene seems a good candidate for intervention studies to elucidate whether a chemoprevention of colon cancer is possible.

Human Intervention Studies

A few studies with conflicting results have been finalized up to now: Greenberg et al., [1994] carried out a clinical trial to test the efficiency of β-carotene, vitamin C and vitamin E in preventing colorectal adenoma. They studied 864 patients who had had an adenoma diagnosed and removed within the previous 3 months. Participants were randomized using a two-by-two factorial design, with the active treatments being β-carotene (25 mg/day) and the combination of 1 g of vitamin C plus 400 mg vitamin E (equivalent to 400 IU). There was no evidence that either β-carotene and/or vitamins C and E reduced the incidence of adenomas. The relative risk for β-carotene was 1.01; for vitamins C and E it was 1.08. The lack of efficacy for supplemental β-carotene persisted when the analyses were restricted to those patients with the lowest quartile of serum β-carotene levels or to those with the lowest quartile of β-carotene intake as reported at enrollment. The finding that β-carotene did not reduce the recurrence of colorectal adenomas is consistent with the results of a smaller trial (n = 291) using a lower dose of 15 mg β-carotene/day [Kikendall et al., 1991].

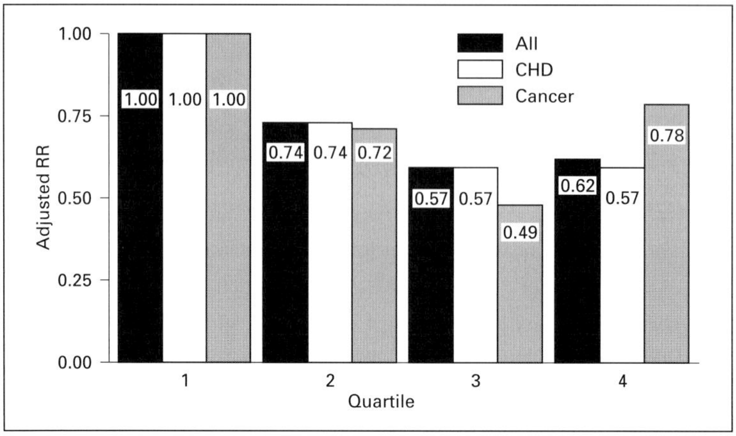

Fig. 2. Mortality rates among patients grouped by plasma β-carotene at entry to the study [Greenberg et al., 1996].

Taken together, β-carotene alone seems not effective to prevent colon cancer in these studies. However, regarding the experimental observation that β-carotene might be effective during early initiation stages it is not surprising that it failed to be chemopreventive in polyp-bearing, high-risk groups. In addition, a lot of different nutrients (fat, fiber, vitamin D, etc.) seem to be critically involved in colon cancerogenesis. The median follow-up period of 8.2 years of the above-mentioned study [Greenberg et al., 1994] showed an inverse relationship between plasma β-carotene levels [Greenberg et al., 1996] (fig. 2). The β-carotene supplementation however revealed no significant effect on mortality from cancer or cardiovascular disease. Taking β-carotene as a 'biomarker' for vegetable intake, it makes more sense to elucidate the preventive effect of vegetables – as long as their real chemopreventive compounds are unexplored – together with other nutrients involved in colon carcinogenesis.

Accordingly, the National Cancer Institute coordinated an adenoma prevention trial (The Polyp Prevention Trial – PPT) involving dietary intervention rather than a nutrient supplement. The study was designed to determine whether a low-fat, high-fiber, vegetable- and fruit-enriched diet would decrease the recurrence rate of large bowel adenomatous polyps. PPT was a multicenter randomized controlled trial examining the effect of a low-fat (20% of total energy intake), high-fiber (18 g/1,000 kcal), vegetable and fruit (5–8 daily servings) dietary pattern on the recurrence of adenomatous polyps of the large bowel, precursors of most colorectal malignancies. 38,277 participants were included and final (T(4)) colonoscopies were completed in early 1998.

Skin Cancer

Epidemiology

Up to now there are no epidemiological data which show that β-carotene or other antioxidative vitamins exclusively prevent skin cancer. Karagas et al. [1997] conducted a nested case-control study of squamous cell skin cancer (SCC) to determine whether the risk was related to plasma concentrations of selenium, α-tocopherol, β-carotene and retinol. The study samples were derived from participants of the Skin Cancer Prevention Study (see section Human Intervention Studies). All participants had at least one basal cell or SCC before study entry. Those who developed a new SCC during the 3- to 5-year follow-up period were selected as cases (n = 132). Controls (n = 264) were chosen at random, from among those who did not develop SCC but were being followed actively at the time the SCC case was diagnosed. No consistent pattern of SCC risk associated with any of the nutrients examined was found. The odds ratios for the highest versus the lowest quartiles of β-carotene, retinol, α-tocopherol and selenium were 0.73, 1.43, 0.89 and 0.86, respectively. From their results the authors follow that their data can be added to the growing body of evidence that these nutrients, at the concentrations evaluated, are not related strongly to SCC risk.

The epidemiological basis to justify an intervention study seems rather weak. There are even few experimental data which show a relationship between UV-induced skin damage, skin cancer and beneficial effects of antioxidants.

Presumed Mechanisms of Action and in vitro Models

Solar UV irradiation results in premature skin aging and is discussed to be an initiating event of skin cancerogenesis [Talwar et al., 1995; Van Weelden et al., 1986]. One reason for premature skin aging is that the UVB-induced expression of matrix degrading metalloproteinases has recently been demonstrated in vivo [Fisher et al., 1996]. Within minutes, low-dose UVB upregulated the stimulators of the metalloproteinase genes [Fisher et al., 1996], the transcription factors AP-1 and NF-κB. Retinoic acid (RA), a transrepressor of AP-1 [Schüle et al., 1991], topically applied to the skin prior to UVB irradiation, substantially reduced the UVB-induced AP-1 activation and metalloproteinase expression. In addition, UVB light induces overexpression of ODC, an enzyme which plays a critical role in carcinogenesis [Niggli and Francz, 1992; Russell, 1985]. The polyamines putrescine, spermidine and spermine have been shown to be essential for mammalian cell growth and function. Intracellular polyamine concentrations are highly regulated by the enzyme ODC (EC 4.1.1.17), which catalyzes the conversion of ornithine to putrescine, the initial and often rate-limiting step in polyamine biosynthesis. The level of ODC activity in quiescent cells is extremely low but readily induced by a wide variety of growth-promoting agents or UV light [Pegg, 1988; Niggli and Francz, 1992]. Rapidly proliferating cells and neoplastic cells express elevated levels of ODC. Inhibition of ODC results in a depletion of putrescine and spermidine pools with the consequence of growth arrest of normal and neoplastic cells in vitro and in vivo [Pegg, 1986; McCann et al., 1987].

Besides the effects on gene expression, carotenoids and in particular β-carotene primarily have antioxidative properties in vitro [Di Mascio et al., 1991; Dix and Aikens, 1993] and in vivo [Reaven et al., 1994]. The provitamin A carotenoids may exert their effects on lipid peroxidation or on gene expression in two ways: (1) as carotenoid or (2) as vitamin A following random or central cleavage. Very recently we were able to show that RA influences UV light-induced lipid peroxidation and ODC activity in human skin fibroblasts [Francz et al., 1998]. One hour postirradiation (p.i.) with 20 J/cm^2 UVA, TBARS production was enhanced by 3 μM atRA treatment (121% of vehicle-treated cells) and decreased by 10 μM atRA treatment (75% of vehicle-treated cells), and not significantly altered in UVB-irradiated cells. Twenty-four hours p.i. with 50 mJ/cm^2 UVB, ODC activity peaked in vehicle-treated cells to 738% of sham-irradiated control cells and was reduced to 493% by 3 μM atRA. Treatment with 10 μM atRA further decreases ODC activity (366%) and this activity peak occurred delayed at 36 h p.i. ODC activity was not significantly enhanced by UVA irradiation (fig. 3). These results suggest that in normal human skin fibroblasts atRA and/or its metabolites influence the UVA generation of ROS by at least two distinct antagonistic mechanisms while the ODC response to UVB-induced DNA damage involves a ROS-independent, retinoid-sensitive regulatory pathway.

The data show that antioxidative effects of β-carotene in human skin might be exerted via formation of RA. Nevertheless, β-carotene and further antioxidative compounds might play an important role in preventing pathological changes of the skin due to UV-induced ROS formation. More than other tissues, the skin is exposed to numerous environmental chemical and physical agents such as UV light causing oxidative stress. In the skin this results in several short- and long-term adverse effects such as erythema, edema, skin thickening, wrinkling and an increased incidence of skin cancer or precursor lesions. However, accelerated cutaneous aging under the influence of UV light, usually termed photoaging, is only one of the harmful effects of continuous oxygen radical production in the skin. Others include cutaneous inflammation, autoimmunological processes, keratinization disturbances and vasculitis.

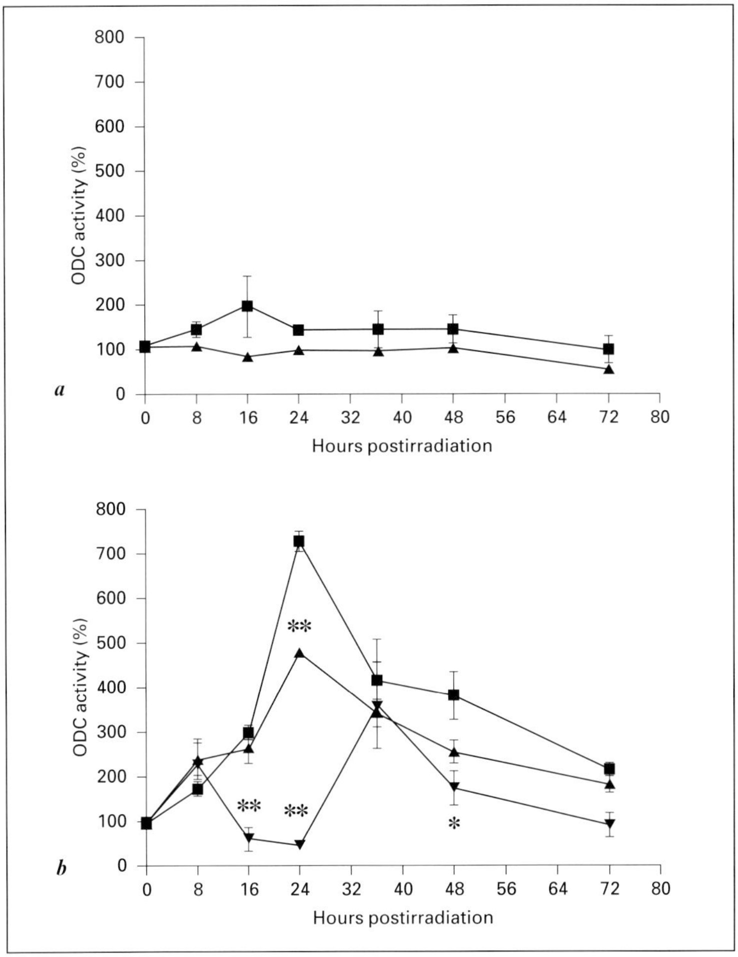

Fig. 3. Effect of atRA on UV-induced ODC response in HFP-1 cells. Cells were treated for 16 h with vehicle alone (■), 3 μ*M* (▲) or 10 μ*M* atRA (▼) before irradiation with 20 J/cm^2 UVA (***a***) or 50 mJ/cm^2 UVB (***b***) and ODC activity (liberation of $^{14}CO_2$ from *L*-[1-^{14}C]-ornithine) determined at the time points postirradiation indicated. Data given are from one representative experiment with three determinations (mean ± SEM) per treatment and time point. ODC activity is expressed as percent activity, with the activity of vehicle-treated, sham-irradiated cells set as 100%. Statistical significance of the difference between vehicle-treated and atRA-treated cells at the confidence level $p<0.05$ (*) or $p<0.01$ (**) [Francz et al., 1998].

Animal Models

Ultraviolet B (UVB, 290–320 nm) exposure results in a variety of cellular insults including induction of cyclobutane pyrimidine dimers in DNA. Accumulation of these lesions can lead to mutations in critical genes and contribute to the development of nonmelanoma skin cancer. α-Tocopherol, which absorbs strongly the UVB, may act as a 'sunscreen'. To explore possible mechanisms of photoprotection, α-tocopherol dispersed in a neutral cream vehicle was topically applied to the dorsal epidermis of female C3H HeNTac mice [Mcvean and Liebler, 1997]. Epidermal DNA from mice receiving UVB for 60 min contained 247 ± 42 pmol thymine dimers/Bmol thymine (2.5 $J/m^2 \cdot s^{-1}$). Topical application of α-tocopherol inhibited dimer formation in a dose-dependent manner. A 1% α-tocopherol dispersion inhibited the formation of thymine dimers to 43% of levels in vehicle controls. Several vitamin E compounds, including α-tocopherol acetate, α-tocopherol methyl ether, γ-tocopherol and δ-tocopherol also inhibited thymine dimer formation, but were 5- to 10-fold less potent than α-tocopherol. From their results the authors suggest that DNA photoprotection is an important mechanism by which topically applied α-tocopherol can inhibit UVB-induced skin cancer. Accordingly, it was demonstrated [Gensler et al., 1996] that neither α-tocopherol acetate nor succinate prevented photocarcinogenesis in a mouse model. In that study, α-tocopheryl acetate or α-tocopheryl succinate not only failed to prevent photocarcinogenesis, but may have enhanced the process. Considering that α-tocopherol esters are included in many skin lotions, cosmetics and sunscreens, further studies are needed to determine the conditions under which topical α-tocopheryl acetate and α-tocopheryl succinate enhance photocarcinogenesis.

β-Carotene as another important antioxidant was tested in different animal models. Santamaria et al. [1986] studied the effect of β-carotene and further dietary carotenoids on benzo(a)pyrene-induced skin cancer in mice. They demonstrated that light-induced formation of ROS leads to an activation of benzo(a)pyrene and subsequently to an increase of skin cancer formations (fig. 4). β-Carotene supplementations resulted in a decrease of skin cancer. This is in agreement with the antioxidant properties of carotenoids which reduce oxidative benzo(a)pyrene activation due to ROS inactivation. The reduction in cancerogenicity of benzo(a)pyrene through carotenoids seems to be an intrinsic function and not due to retinoid formation. This was documented in a further study [Santamaria et al., 1983]. The carotenoids β-carotene and canthaxanthine (CX), with and without provitamin A activity, respectively, when perorally administered to mice, markedly prevent benzo(a)pyrene photocarcinogenic enhancement (BP-PCE), continue to block such BP-PCE and protect significantly against benzo(a)pyrene carcinogenesis in mice maintained in the dark.

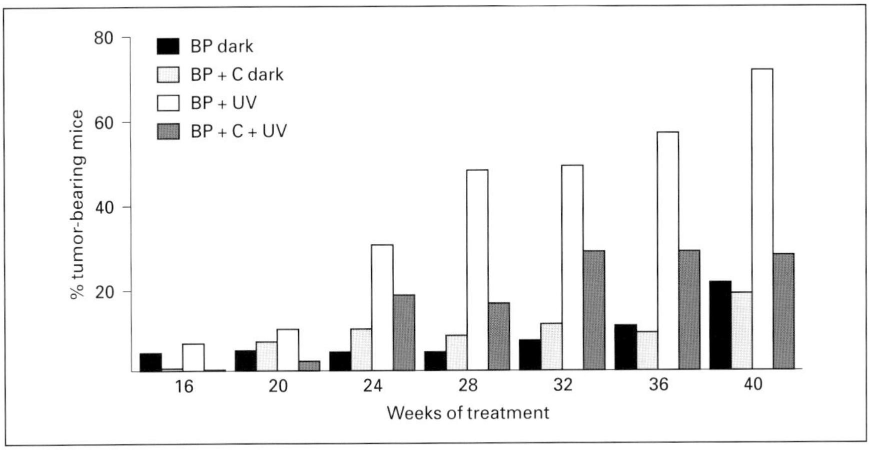

Fig. 4. Mice with tumors following topical treatment with benzo(a)pyrene (BP) with or without β-carotene treatment (C) (4 weeks' pretreatment followed by treatment twice a week). Animals were kept in the dark or during UV irradiation (313 nm for 2 h) during the experiment [Santamaria et al., 1983].

Good evidence that carotenoids per se reduce skin cancer risk comes from studies using non-provitamin A carotenoids. Using mouse skin papilloma as a model, Katsumora et al. [1996] examined whether the antitumorigenic activity of carotenoids was related to their provitamin A activity. Oral administration of CX or β-carotene at 200 mg/kg/day for 14 days in mice significantly reduced the cumulative size of papillomas induced on the skin by 9,10-dimethyl-1,2-benzanthracene ($p<0.05$), after the accumulation of these carotenoids in the tumors. The levels of a protooncogene, c-myc, were simultaneously suppressed in papillomas in carotenoid-treated mice. Because CX cannot be converted metabolically to retinoids, the authors suggest that CX directly inhibited the growth of papillomas. Neither the accumulation of retinoids nor the expression of RA-inducible gene, RA receptor-β, was found in papillomas of CX- and β-carotene-treated mice, suggesting that, like CX, β-carotene might exert the tumor-suppressing effect without being converted to retinoids. Thus a certain antitumorigenic activity of carotenoids appears not necessarily to require provitamin A activity.

Human Intermediate Endpoints

Up to now there are no clear-cut biomarkers predicting the development of skin cancer. Even UV light induces a lot of stress responses in human skin, and these events cannot be taken as reliable biomarkers. Nevertheless, the

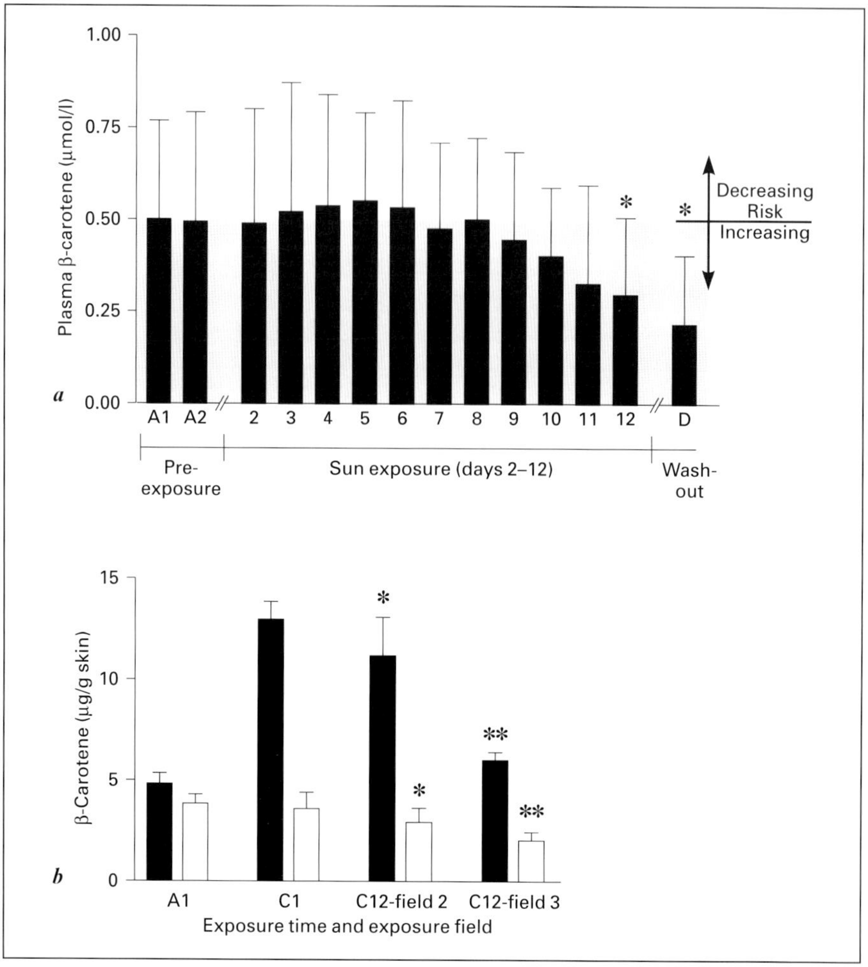

Fig. 5. ***a*** Plasma β-carotene before (A1–A2), during (2–12) and 4 weeks after (D) sun exposure. * Significantly different from 0 ($p < 0.01$). ***b*** Skin β-carotene before (A1) and during sun exposure in supplemented (■) and placebo (□) group. C1 = Start of skin exposure; C12-field 2 = after 12 days' exposure in temporarily exposed skin; C12-field 3 = in continuous exposed skin. * $p < 0.05$, ** $p < 0.01$.

interaction of vitamins with parameters of UV-induced cellular stress response may help to understand the role of these vitamins as photoprotective agents.

UV light reduces plasma [Biesalski et al., 1996] and skin [Gollnick et al., 1996] levels of β-carotene (fig. 5a, b). The decrease of plasma and skin β-carotene as a consequence of sun exposure may have resulted from a direct photodecomposition of β-carotene in the dermal cells and in the capillary bed of the papillary dermis. This photochemical transformation of β-carotene in vivo would be expected to resemble their absorption spectra in organic solvents. Although the major absorption band of carotenoids occurs within the 400- to 500-nm range of the visible spectrum, their absorption spectra extend into the UVA range.

Approximately 35–50% of UVA has been reported to penetrate to the dermis of Caucasians [Everett et al., 1966]. Exposure of epidermis to visible UVA or UVB results in reactions involving singlet oxygen and free radical formation [Dubertret et al., 1982; Mathews-Roth, 1986]. Reactions with peroxyl radicals, generated by UV light, leads to a decoloration of β-carotene [Krinsky and Deneke, 1982; Packer et al., 1981]. Consequently, natural sunlight contributes to a decrease of β-carotene in blood and tissues. The decline of skin β-carotene levels makes the skin more sensitive towards sunlight-induced photodamage. Additionally, UV light can influence the local and systemic immune response, resulting in a decrease of delayed-type hypersensitivity (DTH) and cutaneous hypersensitivity (CHS) reactions or rejection of tumors transplanted in animals [Baadsgaard, 1991; Fuller et al., 1992; Goettsch et al., 1993; Shindo et al., 1994; Stähelin et al., 1984]. Indeed the UV-induced reduction of epidermal Langerhans' cells (LHC), as important local immune cells, is frequently reported. Neale et al. [1997] xamined the effects of chronic and current sun exposure on the number of LHC in epidermal sheets of UV-exposed and unexposed skin of the arms and assessed the effect of sunscreens. Participants were enrolled in a skin cancer prevention trial and had been using sunscreen daily for the previous 3 years. There were significantly fewer LHC on the exposed (463 cells/mm^2 on the unexposed forearm (528 cells/mm^2) ($p < 0.001$). High sun exposure in the previous 2 weeks and a history of predominantly outdoor occupations were both associated with a reduced number of LHC, although age and other biological indicators of chronic exposure were not associated. Sunscreen use was protective against the effects of current but not chronic sun exposure, with a suggestion of a greater effect at higher levels of exposure. Unexpectedly, people with a past history of nonmelanoma skin cancer had more LHC in both the exposed and the unexposed skin. Whether this increase of epidermal LHC is a 'defense' reaction due to formation of skin cancer remains unclear.

An increase of epidermal LHC can be achieved following supplementation of human volunteers with β-carotene [Gollnick et al., 1996]. We conducted a randomized, placebo-controlled, double-blind study in 20 healthy young female students (skin type II + III, body mass index 18–22) to evaluate the efficacy of a moderate dose of 30 mg/d β-carotene after 10 weeks' pre-supplementation and over 13 days of time- and intensity-controlled sunlight exposure at sea level (30° latitude, Red Sea, Eilath, Israel) with regard to development of skin erythema assessed by chromametry at selected skin sites

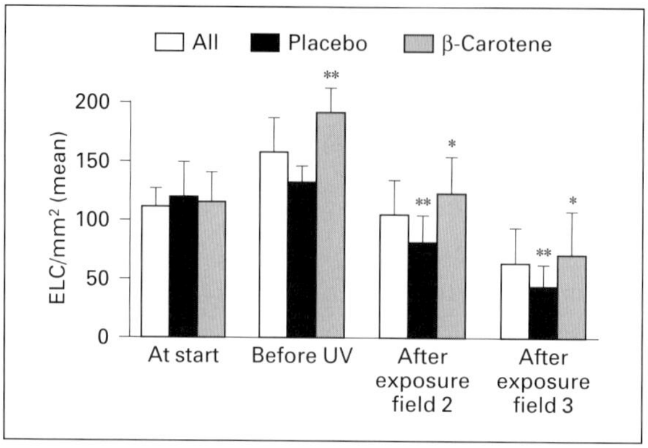

Fig. 6. Epidermal Langerhans' cell (ELC) density at start of the study, before sun exposure (UV) following β-carotene or placebo treatment, after 12 days' exposure in the temporarily (field 2) and continuous (field 3) exposed skin field. $^{*}p<0.05$, $^{**}p<0.01$.

with and without topical UVA/B sunscreen cream. In addition, β-carotene blood levels were regularly checked before and after UV exposure as well as epidermal LHC density by biopsy, DTH by recall antigens and lymphocyte counts by flow cytometry analysis in the peripheral blood.

LHC increased significantly ($p<0.01$) in density per mm^2/epidermis after presupplementation with β-carotene. After UV exposure, LHC density decreased in both groups, however, compared to baseline levels this was significant ($p<0.05$) in the temporary exposed skin region only for the placebo group. The lymphocytic counts and recall antigen profile did not change significantly (fig. 6). Presupplementation with moderate doses of β-carotene before and during natural sunlight exposure combined with topical sunscreens are more effective than sunscreen cream alone.

In addition to the acute deleterious effects of UV light in the sense of erythema and sunburning with initiation of DNA damage, it has been reported several times that natural and artificial UV light, in particular in the UVB range, can adversely influence the local and systemic immune response resulting in a decrease of DTH and CHS reactions or rejections of tumors transplanted in animals [Baadsgaard, 1991; Berne et al., 1984; Fuller et al., 1992; Goettsch et al., 1993; Yoshikawa et al., 1990]. With regard to the skin, the LHC population is dose- and UV wavelength-dependent and is negatively influenced by the sun in numbers and function. The examination of this cell population in the epidermis of the biopsies from our volunteers was also an important parameter to be tested before the start of the study, after the supplementation phase and after UV exposure. Firstly, we could confirm a decrease of cells per mm^2 of epidermis, due to the total cumulative dose of about 10,000 mJ/cm^2 which had reached field 3 at the gluteal region (continuous exposed, non-sunscreen protected). This effect was less pronounced, however, in field 2 (shortly exposed, sunscreen protected), in which at most about a quarter of this UV dose had affected the LHC population. Even in this field the LHC density decreased significantly in the placebo group which is in agreement with a recent report about LHC density decrease after low dose UVB [Murphy et al., 1993]. It is important to note that in the biopsies before UV exposure, the numbers of LHC increased significantly after β-carotene supplementation compared to the baseline and placebo group numbers. Up until now a stimulation has been reported in vitro in murine lymphocytes and Thy-1 cells in the literature [Gollnick and Orfanos, 1991; Schoen and Watson, 1988; Watson et al., 1991]. These results are further supported by other reports that β-carotene in doses higher than 100 mg/day can be immunostimulating, e.g. for T-helper cells, NK cells, Ia expression or increases in T-cell numbers as shown in HIV patients [Coodley et al., 1996]. Therefore, beside the antioxidative capacity of β-carotene, an additional benefit comes from this counteracting effect against the UV-induced alteration of the immune system, e.g. CHS-type insufficiency [Bendich, 1991]. Whereas in the study by Fuller et al. [1992] recall antigen tests showed a decrease in the placebo group but not in the β-carotene-supplemented one, we could neither measure any significant changes in recall antigen response (DTH-type) nor in peripheral blood mononuclear cells.

In another study we estimated the effect of different concentrations of β-carotene (5, 15, 30 mg/day; 8 weeks) on UVB/A irradiation for 14 days (with increasing dose) and skin damage (erythema development, DTH) in a double-blind, placebo-controlled study with 64 female volunteers [Feigenbaum et al., 1997]. The preliminary results clearly show a beneficial effect of β-carotene on UV-induced skin damage with respect to erythema development and DTH.

From these intermediate endpoint studies it can be concluded that β-carotene and further carotenoids may play important preventive roles in human skin. Whether these preventive effects are attributed to cancer prevention should be elucidated in intervention studies.

Intervention Studies

Moon et al. [1997] reported about two randomized clinical chemoprevention trials which began in 1984 to evaluate retinoids in the prevention of skin cancers. Moderate-risk subjects with a history of at least 10 actinic keratoses and at most two prior skin cancers were enrolled in the SKICAP-AK trial and randomized to 25,000 IU retinol or placebo daily for 5 years. High-risk subjects with a risk of at least four prior skin cancers were enrolled in the SKICAP-S/B trial and randomized to receive 25,000 IU retinol, 5–10 mg isotretinoin or placebo daily for 3 years. Data from the SKICAP-AK trial indicate that retinol reduces the incidence of first new squamous cell skin cancers but had no effect on the incidence of first new basal cell skin cancer. The effect of retinoids had no significant benefit on squamous or basal cell skin cancers in the high-risk subjects on the SKICAP-S/B trial, although intervention duration was less than planned. Daily retinol was effective in preventing squamous cell cancers in moderate-risk subjects.

Greenberg et al. [1990] tested the possible cancer-preventing effects of β-carotene by randomly assigning 1,805 patients who had had a recent nonmelanoma skin cancer to receive either 50 mg of β-carotene or placebo per day and by conducting annual skin examinations to determine the occurrence of new nonmelanoma skin cancer. After 1 year the actively treated group's median plasma β-carotene level (3,021 nmol/l) was much higher than that of the control group (354 nmol/l). After 5 years of follow-up, however, there was no difference between the groups in the rate of occurrence of the first new nonmelanoma skin cancer (RR 1.05; 95% confidence interval 0.91–1.22). In subgroup analyses, active treatment showed no efficacy either in the patients whose initial plasma β-carotene level was the lowest quartile or in those who currently smoked. There was also no significant difference between treated and control groups in the mean number of new nonmelanoma skin cancers per patient-year. However, this study does not show a general lack of preventive activity of β-carotene against skin cancer, it shows that in persons with a previous nonmelanoma skin cancer, treatment with β-carotene does not reduce the occurrence of new skin cancers over a 5-year period of treatment and observation.

The study population was at higher risk for developing new skin cancer than a group without any history of former nonmelanoma skin cancer. An 8-year follow-up of this study showed that persons whose initial plasma β-carotene concentrations were in the highest quartile (>0.52 μmol/l) had a lower risk of death from all causes (adjusted RR 0.52) and from cardiovascular diseases (adjusted RR 0.57) compared with persons with initial concentration in the lowest quartile (<0.21 μmol/l). Patients randomly assigned to β-carotene supplementation showed no reduction in relative mortality rates from all causes (adjusted RR 1.03) or from cardiovascular disease (adjusted RR 1.16). There was no evidence of lower mortality following supple- mentation among patients with initial β-carotene concentrations below the median for the study group.

Atherosclerosis

Atherosclerosis and at least its pathological expression, coronary heart disease (CHD) is far more clearly related to dietary factors than cancer. High choles-

Table 1. Stepwise regression analysis of the age-specific IHD mortality

Parameter	r^2	p
Vitamin E	0.62	0.0003
+ Cholesterol	0.79	0.008

terol (with high LDL and low HDL), high triglycerides are generally accepted risk factors for atherosclerosis. High levels of antioxidants however are associated with a lower risk for CHD. The antioxidant vitamins (vitamins C and E) and other protective substances present in fresh and preserved fruits and vegetables and in a host of foods and drinks of vegetable origin, including tea and wine, together, may play a critical role in preventing or delaying the onset of the degenerative diseases, including CHD. Especially one of the antioxidants, α-tocopherol, has been extensively studied and there is a good evidence that vitamin E intake plays a critical and important role in the pathogenesis of CHD.

Epidemiology

In the cross-cultural MONICA project (MONItoring of CArdiovascular disease) has been launched by the WHO to monitor cardiovascular diseases in more than 40 centers over a period of 10 years with the goal to prove the link between risk factors like smoking, cholesterol and high blood pressure with the mortality of ischemic heart disease (IHD). In the complementary vitamin study, the blood plasma levels of lipids, vitamins and carotenoids have been measured in about 100 randomly selected men aged between 40 and 49 years from 16 populations each. The plasma parameters have been correlated with the age-standardized IHD mortality. Surprisingly, the strongest correlation has been observed between vitamin E and the IHD mortality with an r^2 of 0.62 which means that the 7-fold difference of the IHD mortality between the Northern and the Mediterranean countries can be explained by different vitamin E intake by 62%. The stepwise regression analyses revealed cholesterol as the second important parameter that explained an additional 17% of the IHD mortality (table 1) [GEY et al., 1993].

A further category of epidemiological studies are investigations with volunteers where healthy persons are compared with disabled ones. As an example, a study in Scotland will be described [Riemersma et al., 1991]. The hypothesis was tested to prove that risk factors for IHD, like cholesterol, smoking and blood pressure, are already manifest in a early stage of cardiovascular disease, angina pectoris. Since the treatment of angina pectoris includes dietary changes as well, 110 untreated cases have been compared with 394 matched controls. Astonishingly again, the major differences between cases and controls were the plasma vitamin levels, mainly vitamin E, vitamin C and β-carotene, that were inversely correlated with the risk of angina, and vitamin E was the only parameter after adjusting for age, blood pressure, cholesterol, triglycerides, body weight and smoking.

Cohort Studies

This category of studies predicts the forthcoming risk from the analyses carried out at the beginning of the observational period. Three examples will be mentioned: In 1980, investigators in the US analyzed the nutritional habits of 87,245 nurses aged 34–59. At this time, none suffered from cardiovascular disease. During the following 8 years, 115 women died from cardiovascular disease and 437 had a nonfatal myocardial infarction. Comparing the intake of vitamin E (from nutrients and/or from supplements), a significant trend can be observed: Defining the RR of the first quintile = 1 (intake 0.8–2.3 mg vitamin E/day), the risk decreases to 0.74 in the 4th quintile (intake 5.4–14.4 mg/day) with a 95% confidence interval (CI) of 0.57–0.98 after adjusting for age and smoking, and further to 0.66 (95% CI 0.50–0.87) in the 5th quintile (intake 14.5–670 mg/day, median 140). The high vitamin E intakes, mainly in the 5th quintile, originate from supplements. The duration of the supplementation plays an important role: the short-term intake does not show a beneficial effect, however, women who took the vitamin E for more than 2 years benefitted (RR 0.59, 95% CI 0.38–0.91 after adjusting for age, smoking and other risk factors) [Stampfer et al., 1993].

The nutritional habits of 39,910 men working in the healthcare sector in the US were analyzed in 1986. The men were aged between 40 and 75 years and did not suffer from cardiovascular diseases, neither from diabetes nor from hypercholesterolemia. During the following 4 years, 667 cases of cardiovascular disease have been registered. As in the former study, there was a link between the vitamin intake and the cardiovascular risk. Defining the RR of the first quintile = 1 (intake 4.3 mg vitamin E/day), the risk decreased in the 4th and 5th quintile (median of the vitamin E intake 17 and 280 mg/day) to 0.74 (95% CI 0.59–0.93) and to 0.59 (95% CI 0.47–0.75). The corresponding data for β-carotene were: RR = 1 with an intake of 2.4 mg/day; 5th quintile RR = 0.71 (95% CI 0.55–0.92) with an intake of 11.4 mg β-carotene/day. The RR was significantly reduced in men who consumed at least 90 mg vitamin E/day during at least 2 years. The intake of vitamin C was already in the 1st quintile with 92 mg/day above the US recommendation of 60 mg; therefore, the observed trend corresponded to the expectations. In addition, in this study health-conscious persons have been observed whose nutrition is above average [Rimm et al., 1993].

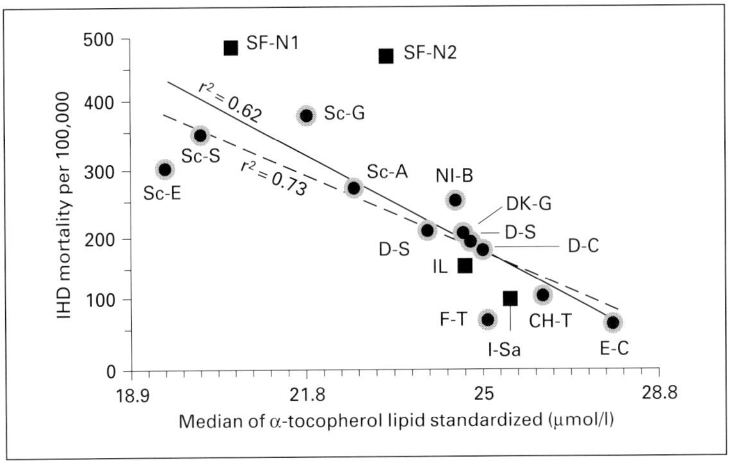

Fig. 7. Lipid standardized vitamin E and CHD mortality [Gey et al., 1991].

In the 3rd study, 34,486 healthy postmenopausal women were questioned about their eating habits in 1986, especially about their consumption of vitamins E, A and C. During the following 7 years, 242 women died from cardiovascular disease. The risk of the disease was inversely correlated with the intake of vitamin E. Unfortunately, there was no question about the duration of the intake of supplements. Therefore, the subgroup analyses of supplement users showing no beneficial effect cannot be interpreted accordingly [Kushi et al., 1996]. In a further study, participants who were told to take vitamin E supplements at two time points exhibited even a lower RR for cardiovascular disease than the ones who indicated the intake only once [Losonczy et al., 1996].

All in all, epidemiological studies point unanimously at a direct link between diet and the risk of cardiovascular disease. Of all analyzed nutritional components, vitamin E shows the most promising inverse correlation with the disease. Nevertheless, epidemiological studies cannot prove any efficacy. They show only possible explanations, the definite prove must be given by intervention studies as they are known from studies with drugs. But here the limits of the feasibility are reached. Thousands of volunteers with an appropriate budget are required to prove a 20% reduction of the mortality risk that would be an enormous progress for the healthcare system. Research is challenged here to find alternatives.

In the WHO/MONICA study, where several European regions were compared, the correlation between cholesterol plasma levels and CHD mortality was rather weak ($r = 0.4$). In contrast, correlation of vitamin E plasma levels and CHD mortality shows a strong correlation ($r = 0.8$) [Gey et al., 1991] (fig. 7). The vitamin E plasma level and CHD mortality were inversely correlated ($p < 0.002$).

Table 2. Vitamin E plasma levels and cardiovascular disease

Group	Population	Endpoint	Vitamin E serum levels, µmol/l	Comments
Gey et al., 1991	North Carelia, Finland Catalonia, Spain	CHD mortality CHD mortality	20.5* 27.5*	481 of 100,000/year 66 of 100,000/year
Riemersma et al., 1991	110 cases 394 controls	Angina risk	22.7 24.0	Angina risk significantly higher in lowest quintile (> 28.2 µmol/l)
Hense et al., 1993	46 cases	Myocardial infarction	33.9 32.8	No difference between cases and controls
Eichholzer et al., 1992	132 cases out of 2,974 men	CHD mortality	First quartile 30.0* Mean 36.0*	No difference between cases and controls

CHD = Coronary heart disease.
* Lipid-adjusted.

Table 2 summarizes studies which deal with a relationship of plasma vitamin E and CHD risk. Two case-control studies [Hense et al., 1993; Eichholzer et al., 1992] did not find a correlation. However, the unexpected high plasma levels (European mean 25 ± 3 µmol/l) may be a result of a randomization error or they can be taken as a hint that all participants have an optimal vitamin E intake.

A few reports are dealing with dietary and supplemental vitamin E intake and CHD risk (table 3).

Despite a reduction of coronary mortality from food-derived vitamin E (62%), Kushi et al. [1996] did not find an association of supplemental use of vitamin E with a significant risk reduction of coronary mortality. However, the authors state that they could not definitively address the effect of vitamin E supplements because they lacked sufficient information about the duration of vitamin E supplement use. However, it is reported from the two largest epidemiologic studies [Stampfer et al., 1993; Rimm et al., 1993] investigating the effect of vitamin E supplements on coronary events that the benefit of vitamin E supplements became obvious only after at least 2 years of use.

Two other non-US-based population studies also found an inverse association between vitamin E status and CHD. One longitudinal study, which included 5,133 Finnish men and women aged 30–69 years who had been initially free of heart disease, [Losconczy et al., 1996; Knekt et al., 1994], reported an inverse association between dietary vitamin E intake and coronary mortality: 32% risk reduction ($p < 0.01$) in the group with the highest vitamin E intake. A Canadian study [DuBroff et al., 1994] in 2,226 men aged 46–76 years reported a significant risk reduction for the first event of IHD in subjects using vitamins, which was strongest for vitamin E supplements.

Table 3. Dietary and supplemental vitamin E intake and CHD risk

Group	Population	Endpoint	Diet effect	Supplement effect
Kushi et al., 1996	21,809 women	Coronary mortality	RR 0.39 (<9.64 IU/day)	None
Losonczy et al., 1996	11,178 elderly	CHD	None	RR 0.59
Knekt et al., 1994	5,133 Finnish men and women	CHD	RR 0.68 (men) (<8.9 IU/day)	Not determined
DuBroff et al., 1994	440 patients	Restenosis rate after PTCA	N.m.	Significantly lower (15.8 vs. 30.7%) in supplement user (<100 IU vitamin E/day)
Hodis et al., 1995	165 men	Progression rate after PTCA	N.m.	Significantly lower in supplement user (<100 IU vitamin E/day)
Stampfer et al., 1993	87,245 female nurses	CHD	None	RR 0.59 (100 IU vitamin E/day over <2 years)
Rimm et al., 1993	39,910 healthcare males	CHD	None	RR 0.54 (100–249 IU vitamin E/day over <2 years)

CHD = Coronary heart disease; N.m. = not mentioned; PTCA = percutanous transluminal coronary angiography; RR = relative risk.

Retrospective analysis of data from clinical trials using coronary angiography as an outcome measure indicated that the use of vitamin E supplements slowed the progression of already established coronary atherosclerosis. A retrospective evaluation of the Cholesterol Lowering Atherosclerosis Study (CLAS) provided evidence that progression of coronary artery lesions, as measured by quantitative angiography, was significantly lower in patients taking vitamin E supplements >100 IU/day [Hodis et al., 1995]. Another retrospective analysis, of 440 patients who underwent a successful coronary angioplasty (follow-up at least 6 months), also showed a significantly lower restenosis rate in patients who took vitamin E supplements: 15.8% in the vitamin E group compared with 30.7% in the nonsupplemented [Stampfer et al., 1993]. Finally, another study reported that the progression of atherosclerosis during 1 year as measured by ultrasound of the carotid artery was significantly lower ($p < 0.04$) in 216 men with vitamin E serum levels ≤ 32.7 µmol/l as compared with those with vitamin E levels ≥ 22.5 µmol/l [Rimm et al., 1993].

Presumed Mechanisms of Action

Vitamin E interferes with two major pathological events which contribute to the early development of CHD: oxidation of LDL and activation of protein kinase C. Table 4 summarizes recent findings. LDL oxidation leads to an increased expression of adhesion factors on the surface of the endothelial cells and

Table 4. Antioxidative and cellular effects of vitamin E

Vitamin E effect	Presumed mechanism	Group
Inhibition of oxidation of plasma lipoproteins and plasma membrane lipids	Antioxidant effect	Esterbauer et al., 1990
Inhibition of monocyte adherence to the endothelium	Reduced E-selectin expression, mechanism not clear	Faruqi et al., 1994
Inhibition of LDL-induced transmigration of monocytes through the endothelium	Reduction of LDL formation with reduced expression of adhesion factors	Navab et al., 1991
Prevention of cytotoxic effects through the endothelium	Antioxidant effect	Hennig et al., 1987
Improvement of vasomotion	1) Protection of EDRF oxidative degradation 2) Inhibition of protein kinase C	Keany et al., 1996
Inhibition of proliferation of smooth muscle cells	Inhibition of protein kinase C	Tasinato et al., 1995
Reduction of ROS formation and liberation from monocytes	Inhibition of protein kinase C	Devaraj et al., 1996

favors the uptake of monocytes into the subendothelial space. In the subendothelial space, blood monocytes are transformed to resident macrophages which accumulate ox-LDL and undergo a conversion to foam cells. Vitamin E which inhibits or reduces formation of ox-LDL might consequently lower foam cell formation and at least atherosclerosis risk. Whereas these early steps of atherosclerosis and the role of vitamin E are generally accepted, the interference of the vitamin with protein kinase C is still controversally discussed.

Very recently we showed that ischemia during aortic aneurysma resection resulted in an assumed leakage of the endothelial barrier with a subsequent loss of vitamin E containing LDL [unpublished data]. 14 days' supplementation with 330 mg vitamin E/day diminished the loss of LDL from the blood during ischemia.

Animal Models

Table 5 summarizes results of animal studies which show a preventive effect of vitamin E and CHD. The data show that vitamin E prevents plaque formation and interferes with smooth muscle cell proliferation and endothelial function. In addition, there are some results which show a dose-dependent vitamin E effect. Feeding 1,000 IU vitamin E/kg food results in a reduction

Table 5. Animal studies with vitamin E for prevention of atherosclerosis

Animal	Induction of atherosclerosis	Diet/duration	α-tocopherol, doses/feed	Goal	Effect on endothelium (compared to control)	Group
Primates (*M. fascicularis*) 6/group	hypercholesterinemia	a) 36 months 0.4% cholesterol ± α-tocopherol b) 12 months 0.4% cholesterol 24 months in addition α-tocopherol	RRR α-tocopherol 108 IU/day	a) Prevention b) Regression of carotis atherosclerosis (ultrasonication)	Carotis stenosis a) Prevention: control = 87% α-tocopherol = 61% b) regression of 33% to 8% (8 months) and 19% (24 months)	Verlangieri et al., 1992
WHHL rabbits 20/group	Hereditary hypercholesterinemia	Standard diet (12 weeks)	all-rac-α-tocopherol (0.5%)	Prevention of atherosclerosis	a) Reduction of atherosclerosis (–32%) b) No difference in storage of cholestorol esters in the aorta	Williams et al., 1992
NZW rabbits 6–10/group	Balloon dilatation (a. iliaca-femoralis); hypercholesterinemia	0.5% cholesterol (9 weeks), then 0.5% cholesterol + α-tocopherol (8 weeks)	all-rac-α-tocopherol (500 mg/kg) + ascorbic acid (500 mg/kg)	Regression and prevention of atherosclerosis	a) No regression b) Prevention of aortic atherosclerosis (lesions –46%, cholesterol esters –40%)	Bocan et al., 1992
NZW rabbits 6–10/group	Hypercholesterinemia	1% cholesterol (28 days)	RRR α-tocopherol a) 1,000 IU/kg b) 10,000 IU/kg	Prevention of endothelial dysfunction	*Doses a)* 1) Prevention of endothelial dysfunction 2) Inhibition of intima proliferation *Doses b)* 1) Increase of endothelial dysfunction 2) Increase of intima proliferation	Keaney et al., 1994
Rats (7/group)	Balloon dilatation (a. carotis); hypercholesterinemia	1% cholesterol	all-rac-α-tocopherol (0.5%)	Prevention of carotis stenosis	Reduction of carotis atherosclerosis and neo-intima proliferation (–30%)	Konneh et al., 1995

of intima proliferation and normalization of endothelial dysfunction (vasodilation) in cholesterol-fed rabbits; in contrast, 10,000 IU/kg food increases endothelial dysfunction and intima proliferation [Keancy et al., 1994].

From animal studies there is good evidence that vitamin E prevents atherosclerosis preferably in risk groups (hypercholesterinemia).

Intermediate Endpoint Studies

In the development of CHD, intermediate endpoints are hard to define. Occurrence of plaques is one endpoint and also angina pectoris can be taken as an endpoint. Whether overexpression of adhesion factors or antibodies against ox-LDL can be taken as intermediate endpoints has to be further elucidated. At the moment, disease-related biomarkers which clearly predict the occurrence of atherosclerosis are missing. Nevertheless, the data of epidemiological and animal studies seem to justify intervention studies of CHD with supplemental vitamin E.

Intervention Studies

Intervention studies are summarized in table 6. The only real intervention study is the CHAOS study.

2,002 patients with angiographically proven atherosclerosis received in a double-blind trial either a placebo (n = 967), 800 IU α-tocopherol (n = 546) or 400 IU α-tocopherol (n = 489) during 510 days (range 3–981). Whereas no significant difference could be observed between the placebo group and the vitamin E group with regard to the cardiovascular death (RR 1.18), the cardiovascular risk was decreased by 47% (RR 0.53) and the nonfatal myocardial infarction by 77% (RR 0.23) (fig. 8). The author did not distinguish between the two vitamin E dosages, since the study was not designed for this purpose.

The α-tocopherol, β-carotene cancer prevention study (ATBC) was designed to prove the efficacy of 50 mg vitamin E, 20 mg β-carotene, or a combination of both for the prevention of lung cancer in smokers. In a subgroup of 1,862 men with a previous infarction, the effect of the supplementation on a secondary event has been analyzed. The fatal cardiovascular episodes were increased in the β-carotene group (RR 1.43) and not influenced by vitamin E. However, the nonfatal myocardial infarction were significantly reduced in the vitamin E group (RR 0.62) (fig. 9). These results are very similar to the outcome of the CHAOS study and should be further elucidated.

There are several studies under way that will add supplementary information about the efficacy of vitamin E. It is noteworthy that in both published intervention trials (ATBC and CHAOS) the vitamin C has not been controlled.

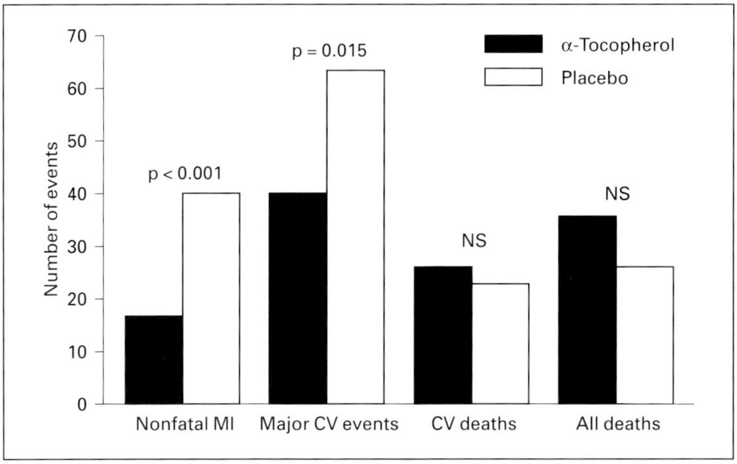

Fig. 8. CHAOS Study: number of cardiovascular events [Stephens et al., 1996].

Table 6. Intervention studies involving vitamin E supplementation and cardiovascular disease

Group	Population	Endpoint	Dose	Comment
DeMaio et al., 1992	100 patients with symptoms of myocardial ischemia	Angiography, thallium and exercise stress test	1,200 IU *d,l*-α-tocopherol for 4 months	Restenosis 35.5% in vitamin E group vs. 47.5% in placebo group Combined incidence of restenosis (angiogram, thallium and exercise test) 34.6% in vitamin E group vs. 50% in placebo group ($p = 0.06$)
ATBC Cancer Prevention Study Group, 1994	29,133 male Finnish smokers	Mortality from IHD	50 IU *d,l*-α-tocopheryl for up to 6 years	602 events in vitamin E vs. 637 in placebo
Rapola et al., 1997	29,133 male Finnish smokers	First occurrence of angina pectoris	50 IU *d,l*-α-tocopheryl acetate for up to 6 years	RR 0.91 ($p > 0.04$) when compared with non-vitamin E group (not significantly difference when compared with placebo)
Stephens et al., 1996	2,002 patients with established CHD	Cardiovascular death and nonfatal myocardial infarction	400 or 800 IU for a median of 510 days	RR 0.23 ($p > 0.001$) for non-fatal myocardial infarction No effect on cardiovascular death
Takamatsu et al., 1995	147 healthy subjects	Alterations in ECG	100 mg *d*-α-tocopheryl acetate for 6 years	Abnormalities in ECG in 7 subjects of the placebo group vs. none in the vitamin E group ($p > 0.02$)

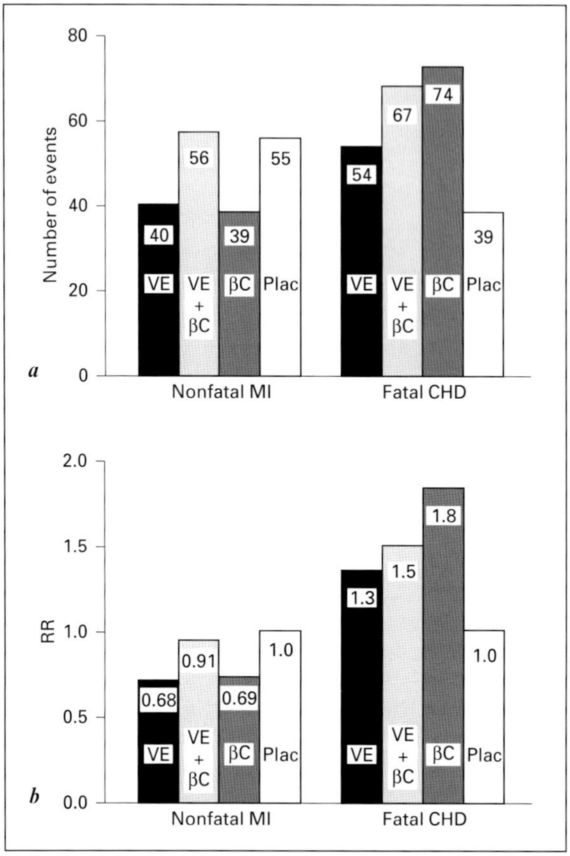

Fig. 9. ***a*** Incidence of major coronary events in men with previous myocardial infarction. ***b*** RR of coronary events in men [Rapola et al., 1997].

Although most data show a protective effect of vitamin E, it is important to pay attention also to the regeneration of the tocopheroxyl radical which can be handled by vitamin C. A sufficient supply of vitamin E has, therefore, to be accompanied by an adequate intake of vitamin C. In a recent study [Schneider et al., 1998] we demonstrated that short-term supplementation with vitamin C and vitamin C plus E has profound and synergistic beneficial effects on DNA damage (fig. 10).

During supplementation with vitamin C (7 days) and vitamin C+E (7 days), a reduction of the micronuclei frequency as a marker for DNA damage was evident in smokers and nonsmokers. However, the decrease was only significant ($p < 0.05$) in smokers following combination of both vitamins. The increase of micronuclei after vitamin washout was significant in smokers

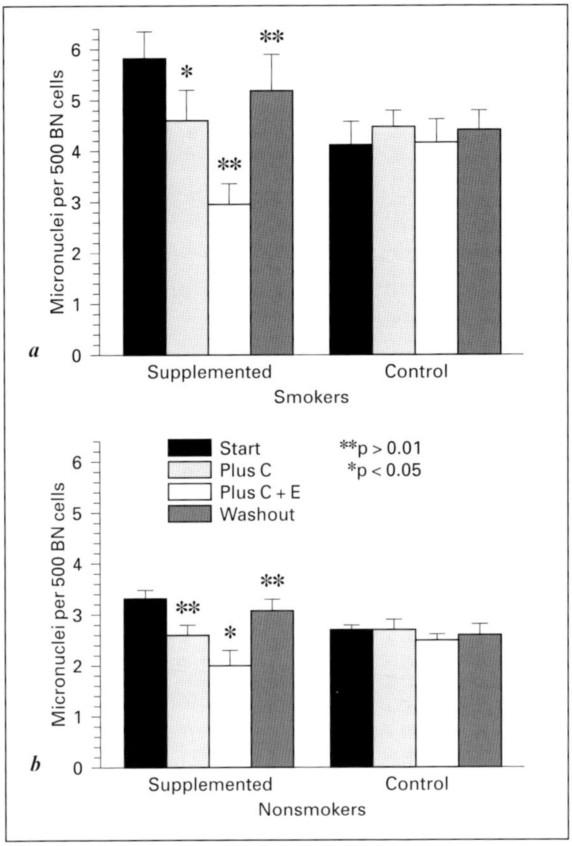

Fig. 10. Micronuclei in blood lymphocytes of smokers (***a***) and nonsmokers (***b***) following vitamin C and E treatment or placebo [Schneider et al., 1998].

($p < 0.05$) as well as in nonsmokers ($p < 0.01$). In addition, there was a significant increase ($p < 0.05$) of the vitamin C radical as measured by means of ESR spectroscopy in supplemented smokers. This shows that an increase of the vitamin C radical may not result in DNA damage or increased lipid peroxidation.

Conclusions

Cancer

The scientific rationale for a justification of an intervention trial as recommended by Omenn is not a sufficient basis for all intervention studies. Consequently, these trials should not have been carried out if the scientific rationale is taken as a prerequisite. With respect to the scientific rationale, especially for those taken from epidemiological studies, it does not seem surprising that there is no evidence from intervention studies that antioxidative vitamins taken as supplements have any beneficial chemopreventive effect in groups at high risk (higher than the mean risk of a healthy population) for lung cancer, colon cancer and skin cancer.

Plasma levels, if not achieved via supplements, should be taken as markers for a specific diet. Consequently, the diet itself is the chemopreventive agent in epidemiological studies and not the 'plasma marker'.

Chemoprevention trials suffer from major problems: (1) Cancer itself is not a reliable endpoint due to its long time from initiation to detectable neoplasma. (2) Intermediate endpoints for precancerous lesions or early cancer do not really exist in 'normal' risk groups which should be the preferred groups for chemoprevention trials. (3) High-risk groups' usual targets in chemoprevention trials might have genetic or metabolic risk factors which cannot be 'chemoprevented'. (4) Bioactive compounds (vitamins, carotenoids, flavonoids, etc.) presumed to be chemopreventive might interact with other bioactive compounds in either a specific ratio or pattern. Only a few of them are available as supplements.

Participants with higher serum β-carotene concentrations at entry to CARET and the ATBC study had fewer subsequent lung cancers, even among those who received the supplements. These results indeed strengthen the benefits of a high dietary intake of fruits and vegetables. A beneficial effect of β-carotene supplementation in ex-smokers [Omenn et al., 1996b] and micronutrient-deficient populations [Blot et al., 1993, 1994] is possible. The ATBC study data show that subjects in the lowest quartile of serum β-carotene at entry (<0.109 μg/ml) had notably elevated lung cancer rates compared with subjects in the second, third and fourth quartiles of serum β-carotene at entry, whose lung cancer rates were similar.

Nevertheless, there are some experimental data and presumed mechanisms of action underlining the biological importance of antioxidative vitamins. However, at the moment these data do not justify an intervention study, especially in high-risk groups. Taken together, all these results do not clearly show that β-carotene alone might have a beneficial effect. Nevertheless, they demonstrate that a diet rich in vegetables contributes to an increase of plasma β-carotene. This is in good agreement with the statement of the WHO Conference on Nutrition and Cancer [Biesalski et al., 1997]. (1) Maintain a 'good' body weight, with a BMI of 20–25. This can be done by controlling energy intake and energy expenditure in recreational or occupational exercise. Obesity is associated with cancer at a number of sites and is not protective for cancer at any site. (2) Eat a diet rich in fruit and vegetables. A high intake is associated with a low risk of cancer at a range of sites (principally in the digestive and respiratory tracts) and is not associated with a high risk of cancer at any site. (3) Eat plenty of whole-grain cereals.

If these recommendations are followed as part of a healthy mixed diet then it will not only help to protect against cancer but also a range of other diseases such as heart disease, atheroma, diabetes, gallstones and hypertension. Consequently, β-carotene is a marker for vegetable intake and this at least will be beneficial. Within all bioactive compounds, present in vegetables, β-carotene might play an important role but at the moment the degree of this importance remains unclear.

Coronary Heart Disease

With respect to CHD and vitamin E, the intervention studies are justified. At present the CHAOS Study has positive results whereas data from ATBC participants are controversial [Rapola et al., 1997, 1998]. However, some large-scale randomized trials of antioxidant vitamins and cardiovascular disease are in progress, including the Women's Health Study [Buring and Hennekens, 1992], the Heart Outcome Prevention Evaluation Study [The Hope Investigators, 1996], and the Heart Protection Study in the United Kingdom. Until the results of these studies become available, there is good reason to believe that a high dose of vitamin E may prevent myocardial infarction in patients with coronary atherosclerosis. For primary prevention, evidence exists that a higher intake of vitamin E will reduce CHD risk.

A recent consensus conference [Biesalski et al., 1997] discussed the state of the art of antioxidant vitamins in prevention and stated that an intake of 15–30 mg vitamin E/day results in 'optimal plasma levels'. Optimal plasma concentrations are 'target parameters', which are currently derived from prospective studies and case studies and from comparisons between countries with large study populations (Basel Study, US Health Professionals' Study, NHANES, Edinburgh Angina Case Study, Vitamin Study of the WHO-MONICA Project). When these threshold levels are reached, the RR of diseases such as CHD and certain neoplastic disorders is low as long as they derive from a suboptimal antioxidant status. The plasma levels resulting from intake of antioxidant vitamins are greatly influenced by additional factors, namely (1) diet (preparation, fat content, type of fats – saturated/unsaturated), (2) homeostatic regulatory mechanisms and (3) other influencing variables such as individual lifestyle or smoking.

With respect to vitamin E, a plasma level of >30 μmol/l (α-tocopherol/cholesterol) is assumed to be optimal.

Taken together, further experimental and intervention trials with selected bioactive compounds or a mixture of different micronutrients are necessary to get more information on how to use these compounds or specific nutrients rich in these compounds for primary or secondary prevention. Nevertheless, an increase of micronutrients, especially vitamins, might have a beneficial effect on cancer risk as documented very recently [Giovannucci et al., 1998]. A higher intake of antioxidant vitamins contributed to a lower risk for UV-induced skin damage and especially vitamin E reduces CHD risk. Whether the 'preventive' doses necessary to ensure long-lasting plasma or tissue concentrations can be achieved by a normal diet or only via supplements or fortified food, remains unclear.

References

Alabaster O, Tang ZC, Frost A, Shivapurkar N: Effect of β-carotene and wheat bran fiber on colonic aberrant crypt and tumor formation in rats exposed to azoxymethane and high dietary fat. Carcinogenesis 1995;16:127–132.

Baadsgaard O: In vivo ultraviolet irradiation of human skin results in profound perturbation of the immune system. Relevance to ultraviolet-induced skin cancer [erratum appears in Arch Dermatol 1991;127:1368]. Arch Dermatol 1991;127:99–109.

Bendich A: Beta-carotene and the immune response. Proc Nutr Soc 1991;54:263–274.

Berne B, Nilsson M, Vahlquist A: UV irradiation and cutaneous vitamin A: An experimental study in rabbit and human skin. J Invest Dermatol 1984;83:401–404.

Biesalski HK, Hemmes C, Hopfenmuller W, Schmid C, Gollnick HPM: Effects of controlled exposure of sunlight on plasma and skin levels of β-carotene. Free Radic Res 1996;24:215–224.

Biesalski HK Editorial: WHO Consensus Conference on Diet and Cancer. Eur J Cancer Prev 1997;6: 315.

Blot WJ, Li JY, Taylor PR, Guo W: Nutrition intervention trials in Linxian, China: Supplementation with specific vitamin/mineral combinations, cancer incidence, and disease-specific mortality in the general population. J Natl Cancer Inst 1993;85:1483–1492.

Blot WJ, Li JY, Taylor PR, Li B: Lung cancer and vitamin supplementation. N Engl J Med 1994;331: 614–614.

Bocan TMA, Mueller SB, Brown EQ, Uhlendorf PD, Mazur MJ, Newton RS: Antiatherosclerotic effects of antioxidants are lesion-specific when evaluated in hypercholesterolemic New Zealand white rabbits. Exp Mol Pathol 1992;57:70–83.

Buring JE, Hennekens CH for the WHSRG. The Women's Health Study: Summary of the study design. J Myocardial Ischaemia 1992;4:27–29.

Cahill RJ, O'Morain CA: Gastric epithelial cell proliferation. Eur J Cancer Prev 1994;3(suppl 2): 55–60.

Chuwers P, Barnhart S, Blanc P, Brodkin CA, Cullen M, Kelly T, Keogh J, Omenn G, Williams J, Balmes JR: The protective effect of β-carotene and retinol on ventilatory function in an asbestos-exposed cohort. Am J Respir Crit Care Med 1997;155:1066–1071.

Coodley GO, Coodley MK, Lusk R, Green TR, Bakke AC, Wilson D, Wachenheim D, Sexton G, Salveson C: β-Carotene in HIV infection: An extended evaluation. AIDS 1996;10:967–973.

Cozzi R, Ricordy R, Aglitti T, Gatta V, Perticone P, De Salvia R: Ascorbic acid and β-carotene as modulators of oxidative damage. Carcinogenesis 1997;18:223–228.

DeMaio SJ, King SB, Lembo NJ, Roubin GS, Hearn JA, Bhagavan HN, Sgoutas DS: Vitamin E supplementation, plasma lipids and incidence of restenosis after percutaneous transluminal coronary angioplasty. J Am Coll Nutr 1992;11:68–73.

Demoly P, Simony-Lafontaine J, Chanez P, Pujol JL, Lequeux N, Michel FB, Bousquet J: Cell proliferation in the bronchial mucosa of asthmatics and chronic bronchitics. Am J Respir Crit Care Med 1994; 150:214–217.

Devaraj S, Li D, Jialal I: The effects of α-tocopherol supplementation on monocyte function. J Clin Invest 1996;98:756–763.
Di Mascio P, Murphy ME, Sies H: Antioxidant defense systems: The role of carotenoids, tocopherols, and thiols. Am J Clin Nutr 1991;53:194S–200S.
Dix TA, Aikens J: Mechanisms and biological relevance of lipid peroxidation initiation. Chem Res Toxicol 1993;6:2–18.
Dubertret L, Santus R, Bazin M, de Sa e Melo T: Photochemistry in human epidermis. A quantitative approach. Photochem Photobiol 1982;35:103–107.
DuBroff RJ, Gretz CA, Sexson RG, Gray WA, White HJ: Vitamin E reduces risk of coronary restenosis. 2nd International Conference. Antioxidant Vitamins and Beta-Carotene in Disease Prevention, Berlin, Oct 10–12, 1994.
Edes TE, Gysbers DG, Buckley CS, Thornton H: Exposure to the carcinogen benzopyrene depletes tissue vitamin A: β-Carotene prevents depletion. Nutr Cancer 1991;15:159–166.
Eichholzer M, Stähelin HB, Gey KF: Inverse correlation between essential antioxidants in plasma and subsequent risk to develop cancer, ischemic heart disease and stroke respectively: 12-year follow-up of the Prospective Basel Study; in Emerit I, Chance B (eds): Free Radicals and Aging. Basel, Birkhäuser, 1992.
Esterbauer H, Dieber-Rotheneder M, Waeg G, Striegl G, Jürgens G: Biochemical, structural, and functional properties of oxidized low-density lipoprotein. Chem Res Toxicol 1990;3:75–92.
Everett MA, Yeargers E, Sayre RM, Olson RL: Penetration of epidermis by ultraviolet rays. Photochem Photobiol 1966;5:533–542.
Faruqi R, de la Motte C, DiCorleto PE: α-Tocopherol inhibits agonist-induced monocytic cell adhesion to cultured human endothelial cells. J Clin Invest 1994;94:592–600.
Feigenbaum A, Hopfenmüller W, Biesalski HK, Gollnick H: Pharmacokinetic of beta-carotene serum levels and recall antigen testing during artificial UVA and UVB/UVA exposure. Arch Dermatol Res 1997;289:293–294.
Fisher GJ, Datta SC, Talwar HS, Wang ZQ, Varani J, Kang S, Voorhees JJ: Molecular basis of sun-induced premature skin ageing and retinoid antagonism. Nature 1996;379:335–339.
Francz PI, Conrad I, Biesalski HK: Effect of retinoic acid on UVA/B-induced gene expression and lipid peroxidation in human skin fibroblasts in vitro. Biol Chem 1998;379:1263–1269.
Frommel TO, Mobarhan S, Doria M, Halline AG, Luk GD, Bowen PE, Candel A, Liao YL: Effect of β-carotene supplementation on indices of colonic cell proliferation. J Natl Cancer Inst 1995;87:1781–1787.
Fuller CJ, Faulkner H, Bendich A, Parker RS, Roe DA: Effect of β-carotene supplementation on photosuppression of delayed-type hypersensitivity in normal young men. Am J Clin Nutr 1992;56:684–690.
Galligan LJ, Jackson CL, Gerber LE: Carotenoids slow the growth of small cell lung cancer cells. Ann NY Acad Sci 1993;691:267–269.
Gensler HL, Aickin M, Peng YM, Xu MJ: Importance of the form of topical vitamin E for prevention of photocarcinogenesis. Nutr Cancer 1996;26:183–191.
Gey KF, Puska P, Jordan P, Moser UK: Inverse correlation between plasma vitamin E and mortality from ischaemic heart disease in cross-cultural epidemiology. Am J Clin Nutr 1991;53:326–335.
Gey KF, Moser UK, Jordan P, Stahelin HB, Eichholzer M, Ludin E.: Increased risk of cardiovascular disease at suboptimal plasma concentrations of essential antioxidants – An epidemiological update with special attention to carotene and vitamin C. Am J Clin Nutr 1993;57:787–797.
Giovannucci E, Stampfer MJ, Colditz GA, Hunter DJ, Fuchs C, Rosner BA, Speizer FE, Willett WC: Multivitamin use, folate, and colon cancer in women in the nurses' health study. Ann Intern Med 1998;129:517–524.
Goettsch W, Garssen J, De Gruijl FR, Van Loveren H: UV-B and the immune system: A review with special emphasis on T-cell-mediated immunity. Thymus 1993;21:93–114.
Gollnick H, Orfanos CE: Theoretical aspects of the use of retinoids as anticancer agents; in Marks R (ed): Retinoids in Cutaneous Malignancy. London, Blackwell Scientific, 1991, pp 41–65.
Gollnick HPM, Hopfenmüller W, Hemmes C, Chun SC, Schmid C, Sundermeier K, Biesalski HK: Systemic beta-carotene plus topical UV-sunscreen are an optimal protection against harmful effects of natural UV-sunlight: Results of the Berlin-Eilath study. Eur J Dermatol 1996;6:200–205.

Greenberg ER, Baron JA, Stukel TA, Stevens MM, Mandel JS, Spencer SK, Elias PM, Lowe N, Nierenberg DW, Bayrd G, et al: A clinical trial of beta-carotene to prevent basal-cell and squamous-cell cancers of the skin. The Skin Cancer Prevention Study Group [erratum appears in N Engl J Med 1991;325: 1324]. N Engl J Med 1990;323:789–795.

Greenberg ER, Baron JA, Tosteson TD, Freeman DH, Beck GJ, Bond JH, Colacchio TA, Coller JA, Frankl HD, Haile RW, Mandel JS, Nierenberg DW, Rothstein R, Snover DC, Stevens MM, Summers RW, Van Stolk RU: A clinical trial of antioxidant vitamins to prevent colorectal adenoma. N Engl J Med 1994;331:141–147.

Greenberg ER, Baron JA, Karagas MR, Stukel TA, Nierenberg DW, Stevens MM, Mandel JS, Haile RW: Mortality associated with low plasma concentration of beta-carotene and the effect of oral supplementation. JAMA 1996;275:699–703.

Hata Y, Kawabe T, Hiraishi H, Ota S, Terano A, Ivey KJ: Antioxidant defenses of cultured colonic epithelial cells against reactive oxygen metabolites. Eur J Pharmacol 1997;321:113–119.

Heilbrun LK, Nomura A, Hankin JH, Stemmermann GN: Diet and colorectal cancer with special reference to fiber intake. Int J Cancer 1989;44:1–6.

Heinenen OP, Albanes D, Virtamo J, Taylor PR, Huttunen JK, Hartman AM, Haapakoski J, Malila N, Rautalahti M, Ripatti S, Maenpaa H, Teerenhovi L, Koss L, Virolainen M, Edwards BK: Prostate cancer and supplementation with α-tocopherol and β-carotene: Incidence and mortality in a controlled trial. J Natl Cancer Inst 1998;90:440–446.

Hennig B, Enoch C, Chow CK: Protection by vitamin E against endothelial cell injury by linoleic acid hydroperoxides. Nutr Res 1987;7:1253–1260.

Hense HW, Stender M, Bors W, Keil U: Lack of an association between serum vitamin E and myocardial infarction in a population with high vitamin E levels. Atherosclerosis 1993;103:21.

Hodis HN, Mack WJ, LaBree L, Cashin-Hemphill LC, Sevanian A, Johnson R, Azen SP: Serial coronary angiographic evidence that antioxidant vitamin intake reduces progression of coronary artery atherosclerosis. JAMA 1995;273:1849–1854.

The Hope Investigators: The HOPE (Heart Outcomes Prevention Evaluation) Study. The design of a large, simple, randomised trial of an angiotensin-converting enzyme inhibitor (ramipril) and vitamin E in patients at high risk of cardiovascular events. Can J Cardiol 1996;12:127–137.

Janne J, Alhonen-Hongleuro L: Inhibitors of ornithine decarboxylase: Biochemistry and applications; in Hayachi S (ed): Ornithine Decarboxylase: Biology, Enzymology and Molecular Genetics. Oxford, Pergamon Press, 1998, pp 7–15.

Jetten AM: Growth and differentiation factors in tracheobronchial epithelium. Am J Physiol Lung Cell Mol Physiol 1991;260:L361–L373.

Jetten AM, Rearick JI, Smits HL: Regulation of differentiation of airway epithelial cells by retinoids. Biochem Soc Trans 1986;14:930–933.

Kaleagasioglu F, Doepner G, Biesalski HK, Berger MR: Antiproliferative activity of retinoic acid and some novel retinoid derivatives in breast and colorectal cancer cell lines of human origin. Arzneimittelforschung. 1993;43:487–490.

Kane KF, Langman MJS, Williams GR: Antiproliferative responses of two human colon cancer cell lines to vitamin D_3 are differentially modified by 9-*cis*-retinoic acid. Cancer Res 1996;56:623–632.

Karagas MR, Greenberg ER, Nierenberg D, Stukel TA, Morris JS, Stevens MM, Baron JA: Risk of squamous cell carcinoma of the skin in relation to plasma selenium, alpha-tocopherol, beta-carotene, and retinol: A nested case-control study. Cancer Epidemiol Biomarkers Prev 1997;6: 25–29.

Kato I, Tominaga S, Matsuura A, Yoshii Y, Shirai M, Kobayashi S: A comparative case-control study of colorectal cancer and adenoma. Jpn J Cancer Res 1990;81:1101–1108.

Katsumura N, Okuno M, Onogi N, Moriwaki H, Muto Y, Kojima S: Suppression of mouse skin papilloma by canthaxanthin and β-carotene in vivo. Possibility of the regression of tumorigenesis by carotenoids without conversion to retinoic acid. Nutr Cancer 1996;26:203–208.

Keaney JF, Gaziano JM, Xu A, Frei B, Curran-Celentano J, Shwaery GT, Loscalzo J, Vita JA: Low-dose α-tocopherol improves and high-dose α-tocopherol worsens endothelial vasodilator function in cholesterol-fed rabbits. J Clin Invest 1994;93:844–851.

Keaney JF, Guo Y, Cunningham D, Shwaery GT, Xu A, Vita JA: Vascular incorporation of α-tocopherol prevents endothelial dysfunction due to oxidized LDL by inhibiting protein kinase C stimulation. J Clin Invest 1996;98:386–394.
Kikendall JW, Mobarhan S, Nelson R, Burgess M, Bowen PE: Oral beta carotene does not reduce the recurrence of colorectal adenomas (abstract). Am J Gastroenterol 1991;36:1356.
Kim PM, De Boni U, Wells PG: Peroxidase-dependent bioactivation and oxidation of DNA and protein in benzo[a]pyrene-initiated micronucleus formation. Free Radic Biol Med 1997;23:579–596.
Knekt P, Reunanen A, Jarvinen R, Seppanen R, Heliovaara M, Aromaa A: Antioxidant vitamin intake and coronary mortality in a longitudinal population study. Am J Epidemiol 1994;139:1180.
Konneh MK, Rutherford C, Li SR, Änggard EE, Ferns GAA: Vitamin E inhibits the intimal response to balloon catheter injury in the carotid artery of cholesterol-fed rat. Atherosclerosis 1995;113: 29–39.
Krinsky IN: Actions of carotenoids in biological systems. Annu Rev Nutr 1993;13:561–587.
Krinsky NI, Deneke SM: Interaction of oxygen and oxy-radicals with carotenoids. J Natl Cancer Inst 1982; 69:205–210.
Kune GA, Kune S: The nutritional causes of colorectal cancer: An introduction to the Melbourne Study. Nutr Cancer 1987;9:1–4.
Kune S, Kune GA, Watson LF: Case-control study of dietary etiological factors: The Melbourne Colorectal Cancer Study. Nutr Cancer 1987;9:21–42.
Kushi LH, Folsom AR, Prineas RJ, Mink PJ, Wu Y, Bostick RM: Dietary antioxidant vitamins and death from coronary heart disease in postmenopausal women. N Engl J Med 1996;334:1156–1162.
La Vecchia C, Decarli A, Fasoli M, Parazzini F, Franceschi S, Gentile A, Negri E: Dietary vitamin A and the risk of intraepithelial and invasive cervical neoplasia. Gynecol Oncol 1988;30:187–195.
Losonczy KG, Harris TB, Havlik RJ: Vitamin E and vitamin C supplement use and risk of all-cause and coronary heart disease mortality in older persons: The established populations for epidemiologic studies of the elderly. Am J Clin Nutr 1996;64:190–196.
Maiani G, Pappalardo G, Ferro-Luzzi A, Raguzzini A, Azzini E, Guadalaxara A, Trifero M, Frommel T, Mobarhan S: Accumulation of β-carotene in normal colorectal mucosa and colonic neoplastic lesions in humans. Nutr Cancer 1995;24:23–31.
Manousos O, Day NE, Trichopoulos D, Gerovassilis F, Tzonou A, Polychronopoulou A: Diet and colorectal cancer: A case-control study in Greece. Int J Cancer 1983;32:1–5.
Mathews-Roth MM: Carotenoids quench evolution of excited species in epidermis exposed to UV-B (290–320 nm) light. Photochem Photobiol 1986;43:91–93.
McCann PP, Pegg AE, Sjoerdsma A: Inhibition of polyamine metabolism; in Biological Significance and Basis for New Therapies. Orlando, Academic Press, 1987, pp 1–371.
McLarty JW, Holiday DB, Girard WM, Yanagihara RH, Kummet TD, Greenberg SD: Beta-carotene, vitamin A and lung cancer chemoprevention: Results of an intermediate endpoint study. Am J Clin Nutr 1995;62:1431S–1438S.
McVean M, Liebler DC: Inhibition of UVB-induced DNA photodamage in mouse epidermis by topically applied alpha-tocopherol. Carcinogenesis 1997;18:1617–1622.
Moon TE, Levine N, Cartmel B, Bangert JL: Retinoids in prevention of skin cancer. Cancer Lett 1997; 114:203–205.
Morabia A, Sorenson A, Kumanyika SK, Abbey H, Cohen BH, Chee E: Vitamin A, cigarette smoking and airway obstruction. Am Rev Respir Dis 1989;140:1312–1316.
Morabia A, Menkes MJ, Comstock GW, Tockman MS: Serum retinol and airway obstruction. Am J Epidemiol 1990;132:77–82.
Murata T, Tamai H, Morinobu T, Manago M: Effect of long-term administration of beta-carotene on lymphocyte subsets in humans. Am J Clin Nutr 1994;60:597–602.
Murphy GM, Norris PG, Young AR, Corbett MF, Hawk JL: Low-dose ultraviolet-B irradiation depletes human epidermal Langerhans' cells. Br J Dermatol 1993;129:674–677.
Navab M, Imes SS, Hama SY, Hough GP, Ross LA, Bork RW, Valente AJ, Berliner JA, Drinkwater DC, Laks H, Fogelman AM: Monocyte transmigration induced by modification of low-density lipoprotein in cocultures of human aortic wall cells is due to induction of monocyte chemotactic protein 1 synthesis and is abolished by high-density lipoprotein. J Clin Invest 1991;88:2039–2046.

Neale R, Russell A, Muller HK, Green A: Sun exposure, sunscreen and their effects on epidermal Langerhans' cells. Photochem Photobiol 1997;66:260–264.
Niggli HJ, Francz PI: May ultraviolet light-induced ornithine decarboxylase response in mitotic and post-mitotic human skin fibroblasts serve as a marker of aging and differentiation? Age 1992;15:55–60.
Nomura AM, Stemmermann GN, Heilbrun LK, Salkeld RM, Vuilleumier JP: Serum vitamin levels and the risk of cancer of specific sites in men of Japanese ancestry in Hawaii. Cancer Res 1985;45:2369–2372.
O'Brien TG, Simsiman RC, Boutwell RK: Induction of the polyamine-biosynthetic enzymes in mouse epidermis by tumor-promoting agents. Cancer Res 1975;35:1662–1670.
Omenn GS, Goodman GE, Thornquist MD, Balmes J, Cullen MR, Glass A, Keogh JP, Meyskens FL Jr, Valanis B, Williams JH Jr, Barnhart S, Cherniack MG, Brodkin CA, Hammar S: Risk factors for lung cancer and for intervention effects in CARET, the beta-carotene and retinol efficacy trial. J Natl Cancer Inst 1996a;88:1550–1559.
Omenn GS, Goodman GE, Thornquist MD, Balmes J, Cullen MR, Glass A, Keogh JP, Meyskens FL Jr, Valanis B, Williams JH Jr, Barnhart S, Hammar S: Effects of a combination of beta-carotene and vitamin A on lung cancer and cardiovascular disease. N Engl J Med 1996b;334:1150–1155.
Packer JE, Mahood JS, Mora-Arellano VO, Slater TF, Willson RL, Wolfenden BS: Free radicals and singlet oxygen scavengers: Reaction of a peroxy-radical with beta-carotene, diphenyl furan and 1,4-diazobicyclo(2,2,2)-octane. Biochem Biophys Res Commun 1981;98:901–906.
Paiva SAR, Godoy I, Vannucchi H, Fávaro RMD, Geraldo RRC, Campana AO: Assessment of vitamin A status in chronic obstructive pulmonary disease patients and healthy smokers. Am J Clin Nutr 1996;64:928–934.
Pegg AE: Recent advances in the biochemistry of polyamines in eukaryotes. Biochem J 1986;234:249–262.
Pegg AE: Polyamine metabolism and its importance in neoplastic growth and a target for chemotherapy. Cancer Res 1988;48:759–774.
Phillips RW, Kikendall JW, Luk GD, Willis SM, Murphy JR, Maydonovitch C, Bowen PE, Stacewicz-Sapuntzakis M, Wong RKH: β-Carotene inhibits rectal mucosal ornithine decarboxylase activity in colon cancer patients. Cancer Res 1993;53:3723–3725.
Potter JD, McMichael AJ: Diet and cancer of the colon and rectum: A case-control study. J Natl Cancer Inst 1986;76:557–569.
Princen HMG, Van Poppel G, Vogelezang C, Buytenhek R, Kok FJ: Supplementation with vitamin E but not β-carotene in vivo protects low density lipoprotein from lipid peroxidation in vitro: Effect of cigarette smoking. Arterioscler Thromb 1992;12:554–562.
Rapola JM, Virtamo J, Ripatti S, Huttunen JK, Albanes D, Taylor PK, Heinonen OP: Randomized trial of α-tocopherol and β-carotene supplements on incidence of major coronary events in men with previous myocardial infarction. Lancet 1997;349:1715–1720.
Rapola JM, Virtamo J, Ripatti S, Haukka JK, Huttunen JK, Albanes D, Taylor PR, Heinonen OP: Effects of α-tocopherol and β-carotene supplements on symptoms, progession, and prognosis of angina pectoris. Heart 1998;79:454–458.
Reaven PD, Ferguson E, Navab M, Powell FL: Susceptibility of human LDL to oxidative modification: Effects of variations in β-carotene concentration and oxygen tension. Arterioscler Thromb 1994;14:1162–1169.
Riemersma RA, Wood DA, MacIntyre CC, Elton RA, Gey KF, Oliver MF: Risk of angina pectoris and plasma concentrations of vitamin A vitamin C and vitamin E and carotene. Lancet 1991;337:1–5.
Rimm EB, Stampfer MJ, Ascherio A, Giovannucci E, Colditz GA, Willett WC: Vitamin-E consumption and the risk of coronary heart disease in men. N Engl J Med 1993;328:1450–1456.
Russell DH: Ornithine decarboxylase as a marker of carcinogenesis; in Milman HA, Weisburger EK (eds): Handbook of Carcinogene Testing. Park Ridge, Noyes, 1985, pp 464–481.
Santamaria L, Bianchi A, Arnaboldi A, Andreoni L, Bermond P: Dietary carotenoids block photocarcinogenic enhancement by benzo(a)pyrene and inhibit its carcinogenesis in the dark. Experientia 1983; 39:1043–1045.
Santamaria L, Bianchi A, Arnaboldi A, Andreoni L, Santagati G, Ravetto C, Bianchi L, Pizzala R, Bermond P: Supplemental carotenoids prevent skin cancer by benzo(a)pyrene, breast cancer by PUVA, and gastric cancer by MNNG. Relevance in human chemoprevention; in Meyskens FL Jr, Prasad KN (eds): Vitamins and Cancer. Human Cancer Prevention by Vitamins and Micronutrients. Clifton, Humana Press, 1986, pp 139–159.

Schneider M, Diemer K, Engelhart K, Zankl H, Trommer WE, Biesalski HK: Protective effects of vitamin C and E in smokers monitored by ascorbyl radical formation in plasma and the frequency of micronuclei in lymphocytes. Free Radic Res 2000 (in press).

Schoen DJ, Watson RR: Prevention of UV irradiation-induced suppression of monocyte functions by retinoids and carotenoids in vitro. Photochem Photobiol 1988;48:659–663.

Schüle R, Rangarajan P, Yang N, Kliewer S, Ransone LJ, Bolado J, Verma IM, Evans RM: Retinoic acid is a negative regulator of AP-1 responsive genes. Proc Natl Acad Sci USA 1991;88:6092–6096.

Shindo Y, Witt E, Han D, Packer L: Dose-response effects of acute ultraviolet irradiation on antioxidants and molecular markers of oxidation in murine epidermis and dermis. J Invest Dermatol 1994;102: 470–475.

Shivapurkar N, Tang Z, Frost A, Alabaster O: Inhibition of progression of aberrant crypt foci and colon tumor development by vitamin E and β-carotene in rats on a high-risk diet. Cancer Lett 1995;91: 125–132.

Stähelin HB, Rosel F, Buess E, Brubacher G: Cancer, vitamins, and plasma lipids: Prospective Basel Study. J Natl Cancer Inst 1984;73:1463–1468.

Stampfer MJ, Hennekens CH, Manson JE, Colditz GA, Rosner B, Willett WC: Vitamin-E consumption and the risk of coronary heart disease in men. N Engl J Med 1993;328:1450–1456.

Stephens NG, Parsons A, Schofield PM, Kelly F, Cheeseman K, Mitchinson MJ, Brown MJ: Randomised controlled trial of vitamin E in patients with coronary disease: Cambridge Heart Antioxidant Study (CHAOS). Lancet 1996;347:781–786.

Stich HF, Rosin MP, Vallejera MO: Reduction with vitamin A and beta-carotene administration of proportion of micronucleated buccal mucosal cells in Asian betal nut and tobacco chewers. Lancet 1984;i: 1204–1206.

Stofft E, Biesalski HK, Zschaebitz A, Weiser H: Morphological changes in the tracheal epithelium of guinea pigs in conditions of 'marginal' vitamin A deficiency. Int J Vitam Nutr Res 1991;62:134–142.

Takamatsu S, Takamatsu M, Satoh K, Imaizumi T, Yoshida H, Hiramoto M, Koyama M, Ohgushi Y, Mizuno S: Effects on health of dietary supplementation with 100 mg *d*-alpha-tocopheryl acetate, daily for 6 years. J Int Med Res 1995;23:342–357.

Talwar HS, Griffiths CE, Fisher GJ, Hamilton TA, Voorhees JJ: Reduced type I and type III procollagens in photodamaged adult human skin. J Invest Dermatol 1995;105:285–290.

Tang G, Shiau A, Russell RM, Mobarhan S: Serum retinoic acid levels in patients with resected benign and malignant colonic neoplasias on β-carotene supplementation. Nutr Cancer 1995;23:291–298.

Tasinato A, Boscoboinik D, Bartoli GM, Maroni P, Azzi A: *d*-α-Tocopherol inhibition of smooth muscle cell proliferation occurs at physiological concentrations, correlates with protein kinase C inhibition, and is independent of its antioxidant properties. Proc Natl Acad Sci USA 1995;92:12190–12194.

The Alpha-Tocopherol, Beta Carotene Cancer Prevention Study Group: The effect of vitamin E and beta-carotene on the incidence of lung cancer and other cancers in male smokers. N Engl J Med 1994; 330:1029–1035.

Tuyns AJ: A case-control study on colorectal cancer in Belgium. Preliminary results. Soz Praventivmed 1986;31:81–82.

Tuyns AJ, Riboli E, Doornbos G, Pequignot G: Diet and esophageal cancer in Calvados (France). Nutr Cancer 1987;9:81–92.

Van Poppel G, Goldbohm RA: Epidemiologic evidence for beta-carotene and cancer prevention. Am J Clin Nutr 1995;62:1393S–1402S.

Van Weelden H, De Gruijl FR, Van der Leun JC, Urbach F, Gange RW (eds): The Biological Effects of UV-A Radiation. New York, Praeger, 1986, pp 137–146.

Verlangieri AJ, Bush MJ: Effects of *d*-α-tocopherol supplementation on experimentally induced primate atherosclerosis. J Am Coll Nutr 1992;11:131–138.

Verma AK: Inhibition of tumor promotion by *DL*-alpha-difluoromethylornithine, a specific irreversible inhibitor of ornithine decarboxylase. Basic Life Sci 1990;52:195–204.

Wang XD, Krinsky NI, Tang GW, Russell RM: Retinoic acid can be produced from excentric cleavage of beta-carotene in human intestinal mucosa. Arch Biochem Biophys 1992;293:298–304.

Watson RR, Prabhala RH, Plezia PM, Alberts DS: Effect of beta-carotene on lymphocyte subpopulations in elderly humans: Evidence for a dose-response relationship. Am J Clin Nutr 1991;53:90–94.

Weimann BJ, Weiser H: Functions of vitamin E in reproduction and in prostacyclin and immunoglobulin synthesis in rats. Am J Clin Nutr 1991;53:1056S–1060S.
Williams RJ, Motteram JM, Sharp CH, Gallagher PJ: Dietary vitamin E and the attenuation of early lesion development in modified Watanabe rabbits. Atherosclerosis 1992;94:153–159.
Wolterbeek APM, Roggeband R, Van Moorsel CJA, Baan RA, Koeman JH, Feron VJ, Rutten AAJJL: Vitamin A and β-carotene influence the level of benzo[*a*]pyrene-induced DNA adducts and DNA-repair activities in hamster tracheal epithelium in organ culture. Cancer Lett 1995;91:205–214.
Yoshikawa T, Rae V, Bruins-Slot W, Van den Berg JW, Taylor JR, Streilein JW: Susceptibility to effects of UVB radiation on induction of contact hypersensitivity as a risk factor for skin cancer in humans. J Invest Dermatol 1990;95:530–536.
Zhang LX, Cooney RV, Bertram JS: Carotenoids enhance gap junctional communication and inhibit lipid peroxidation in C3H/10T1/2 cells: Relationship to their cancer chemopreventive action. Carcinogenesis 1991;12:2109–2114.

Prof. Hans K. Biesalski, University Hohenheim, Department of Biological Chemistry and Nutrition, Fruwirthstrasse 12, D–70593 Stuttgart (Germany)
Tel. +49 711 459 3611, Fax +49 711 459 3822, E-Mail biesal@uni_hohenheim.de

Walter P, Hornig D, Moser U (eds): Functions of Vitamins beyond Recommended Dietary Allowances. Bibl Nutr Dieta. Basel, Karger, 2001, No 55, pp 135–147

Mechanisms of Vitamin-Mediated Anti-Inflammatory and Immunomodulatory Activity

Ronald Anderson

Medical Research Council Unit for Inflammation and Immunity, Department of Immunology, Institute for Pathology, University of Pretoria, South Africa

Optimum functioning of the human immune system is inextricably linked to the nutritional status of the host. With respect to vitamins, adequate intake of vitamins A, B_6, C, E and possibly D appears to be necessary for the maintenance of effective host defences against microorganisms and viruses. In addition, vitamins C and E have potentially important anti-inflammatory, cytoprotective properties which enable the cellular components of the host immune system to function efficiently in the setting of minimal tissue damage.

Vitamins and Host Immunodefences

The human immunodefence system is extremely well-ordered and highly specialized for the efficient performance of its primary function, which is to protect the host against the unremitting threat to health and survival posed by environmental microbial and viral pathogens. To counter this threat, Nature has evolved an intricate, but remarkably effective network of interacting cellular immunodefences. Strategic placement, vigilance, reserve capacity and amplification potential are key features of the human immune system, enabling rapid and efficient mobilization of its cellular effector mechanisms. Given the reserve capacity inherent in these cellular immune effector mechanisms, it is probable, however, that only prolonged vitamin deficiency states predispose to an increased frequency of infective episodes. Exceptions to this are the very young and the elderly, who have age-related immune dysfunction, as well as individuals infected with the human immunodeficiency virus (HIV).

Table 1. Vitamins which may promote optimum immune functions in humans

Vitamins	Immunomodulatory activities
Vitamin A	Maintenance of epithelial integrity; efficient production of antibodies to T-dependent microbial and viral antigens
Vitamin B_6	Maturation and optimum function of T lymphocytes
Vitamin C	Promotes efficient chemotaxis of phagocytes, particularly neutrophils, and may augment cell-mediated immunity
Vitamin D	May be necessary for acquisition of mycobactericidal and tumouricidal activity by macrophages
Vitamin E	Augments T-lymphocyte and macrophage functions

Vitamin A, several of the B vitamins (riboflavin, pantothenic acid and especially pyridoxine), vitamin C, vitamin E and possibly vitamin D promote optimum protective host immune responses. The antioxidative vitamins, C and E, also neutralize pro-inflammatory, cytotoxic-reactive oxidants and bioactive phospholipids generated as by-products of activation of cellular defence systems. These anti-inflammatory properties of vitamins C and E are of potential importance in the prevention of degenerative diseases and cancer.

The vitamins reviewed here (A, B_6, C, D and E) are those for which convincing evidence of beneficial immunomodulatory effects in humans have been described. These are summarized in table 1. Vitamin B_{12} and folic acid, which primarily affect haematopoiesis, have not been included.

Vitamin A

Mild deficiency of vitamin A, which is common in developing countries, increases the severity of childhood infectious diseases, especially diarrhoea and measles, and associated mortality [1]. Correction of this deficiency has resulted in reductions in mortality ranging from 20 to 50% in the groups that received vitamin A by comparison with the corresponding placebo groups. Vitamin A deficiency during pregnancy may be associated with increased transmission of HIV from mother to child [2], while vitamin A supplementation of infants born to HIV-infected mothers is accompanied by a significant reduction in overall morbidity and mortality, as well as decreases of 77 and 49% for hospital admissions and all diarrhoea respectively [3]. The exact mechanisms by which vitamin A protects children against infectious diseases have not been conclusively established. However, evidence from clinical studies, as well as from animal models of experimental infection in the setting of hypovitaminosis A, suggest that deficiency of this vitamin may compromise the production of specific antibodies, especially those of the IgG1 and IgG3 subclasses, against T-lymphocyte-dependent antigens.

Administration of vitamin A to children hospitalized with severe measles, and who had no clinical signs of vitamin A deficiency, has been reported to result in accelerated recovery, a marked reduction in morbidity, and a significant increase in the serum concentrations of measles IgG antibody [4]. In other studies, also conducted in developing countries, vitamin A supplementation of children aged 6 months or older at the same time as immunization, in accordance with a WHO recommendation, resulted in significantly increased levels of circulating specific IgG antibodies following administration of measles vaccine [5] or tetanus toxoid [6].

In a mouse model of experimental infection, hypovitaminosis A was accompanied by dramatically decreased production of specific antibodies of the IgG1 and IgG3 subclasses to microbial pathogens [7], while the primary IgG responses of vitamin A-deficient rats immunized with a series of T-cell-dependent microbial antigens, but not those elicited by T-cell-independent antigens, were markedly reduced [8]. In both cases repletion with vitamin A or its derivatives restored these defective IgG responses [7, 8]. While vitamin A may also potentiate the functions of macrophages and cytotoxic T lymphocytes [8], the aforementioned findings suggest that vitamin A primarily promotes optimum protective antibody responses, particularly those of the IgG1 and IgG3 subclasses, to T-cell-dependent microbial and viral antigens.

Although the exact biochemical/molecular mechanisms of vitamin A-mediated immunopotentiation remain to be established, Cantorna et al. [9] have reported that vitamin A deficiency causes a T-helper cell imbalance in mice experimentally infected with the nematode, *Trichinella spiralis*. This was characterized by a strong Th1 cell response at the expense of the Th2 cell response, which was opposite to the T-helper cell responses of control mice. Th1 cells secrete cytokines which promote cell-mediated immune responses, while cytokines produced by Th2 cells drive antibody synthesis, including production of those of the IgG1 and IgG3 subclasses. In vitamin A-deficient animals, the defective Th2 cell responses were associated with hypersecretion of the Th1-derived cytokine γ-interferon, resulting in suppression of the Th2 cytokines which drive clonal expansion of B lymphocytes. Addition of retinoic acid to T-lymphocyte cultures from the vitamin A-deficient mice was accompanied by reduced synthesis of γ-interferon, and increased frequency of Th2 cells, and restoration of the Th1-Th2 balance [9]. The authors concluded that vitamin A, following transformation to retinoic acid, binds to nuclear receptors which regulate cytokine gene expression in T cells, favouring development of Th2 cells and antibody synthesis [9].

Maintenance of epithelial integrity, probably by regulation of cellular differentiation at the level of nuclear receptors, is an additional mechanism by which vitamin A sustains host defences, probably by preventing adherence and penetration of micro-organisms and viruses, as well as by optimizing leukocyte trafficking on and across the epithelium [10]. Interestingly, loss of ciliae from ciliated respiratory epithelium has been reported to precede the development of squamous metaplasia in vitamin A-deficient guinea pigs [11]. However there are no studies in human subjects which have addressed the effects of hypovitaminosis A on the functions (ciliary beating, mucociliary clearance) and structural integrity of ciliated respiratory epithelium.

Vitamin B_6

Severe experimentally induced deficiency of vitamin B_6 in laboratory animals is primarily associated with defective intrathymic maturation and functions of T lymphocytes [12–14]. In elderly humans, marginal deficiency of this vitamin is accompanied by secondary immunodeficiency, which is characterized by decreased numbers and proliferative activities of circulating T lymphocytes, as well as diminished production of interleukin-2 by these cells. These abnormalities are corrected by short-term administration of vitamin B_6 at a dose of 50 mg/day [13, 14]. The exact biochemical/molecular mechanisms by which vitamin B_6 promotes optimum function of T lymphocytes remain to be established. However, the cofactor requirement for this vitamin by multiple enzymes suggest that numerous T-lymphocyte metabolic pathways may be involved.

Vitamin D

Although definitive proof remains outstanding, it has been proposed that hypovitaminosis D compromises host defences against *Mycobacterium tuberculosis* [15] and predisposes to the development and progression of carcinomas of the breast, prostate and colon [16].

In the case of tuberculosis, it has been reported that vitamin D augments the antimycobacterial activity of human monocytes in vitro [15]. Exposure to γ-interferon or bacterial endotoxin induces 1-hydroxylase activity in these cells, enabling synthesis of $1,25(OH)_2D_3$ [15]. Exposure of monocytes to physiologically relevant concentrations of this agent in vitro promotes differentiation of these cells and acquisition of mycobacteriocidal activity. While this apparent autocrine activation of monocytes is a potentially important mechanism of immune-mediated eradication of *M. tuberculosis*, its clinical relevance remains to be established [17], as does the predisposing role of hypovitaminosis D in the development of pulmonary tuberculosis.

Data from experimental systems and a limited number of epidemiological studies appear to support the hypothesis that sunlight-generated vitamin D_3

derivatives contribute to a lower incidence of the clinically-apparent forms of breast, prostate and colon cancer [16]. These agents, especially $1,25(OH)_2D_3$, have been reported to induce the differentation of several neoplastic cell types and to arrest or retard their proliferation in vitro, while acting as chemopreventive agents in animal models of experimental cancer chemotherapy [16]. These beneficial anticancer properties of vitamin D are probably mediated at the nuclear level via the interaction of $1,25(OH)_2D_3$ with the vitamin D receptor, the complex then acting as a transcription factor that modulates the activity of a number of human genes, including those that regulate cellular growth and differentiation [18].

In addition, $1,25(OH)_2D_3$ may also activate host antitumour defences by at least two distinct mechanisms. Firstly, as described above, exposure of monocytes to $1,25(OH)_2D_3$ may promote differentation of these cells with consequent acquisition of tumouricidal activity [16]. A second potential mechanism has been described by Young et al. [19] who reported that certain types of tumour produce the cytokine, granulocyte-macrophage colony-stimulating factor (GM-CSF), which in turn inactivates tumour-directed host defences by inducing the production of a poorly defined, bone marrow-derived suppressor cell. Treatment of tumour tissue with $1,25(OH)_2D_3$ in combination with γ-interferon resulted in inhibition of the production of GM-CSF and augmentation of antitumour immunity, which was characterized by expansion and activation of tumour infiltrating $CD8^+$ T lymphocytes [19].

Vitamin C and Host Defences

Because of its ability to function efficiently as a scavenger of reactive oxidants in both the extracellular and intracellular compartments, vitamin C appears to play an important role in host defence against microbial pathogens. Augmentation of host defences is achieved by protection of phagocytes, particularly neutrophils, against auto-oxidative dysfunction [reviewed in 20]. Reactive oxidants, which are produced in abundance by activated phagocytes, are not only potent, albeit indiscriminate, antimicrobial agents, but are also autotoxic to these cells, causing inactivation of various cellular functions, especially chemotaxis [20]. Hypovitaminosis C in both animals and humans is accompanied by auto-oxidative inhibition of neutrophil migration and increased frequency and/or severity of bacterial infections [20–22]. Hypochlorous acid (HOCl), which is produced in large quantities by activated neutrophils, and which is efficiently neutralized by vitamin C, is a particularly potent mediator of auto-oxidative inactivation of leukocyte migration. This permeant reactive oxidant inhibits the activity of the oxidation-sensitive, cytosolic,

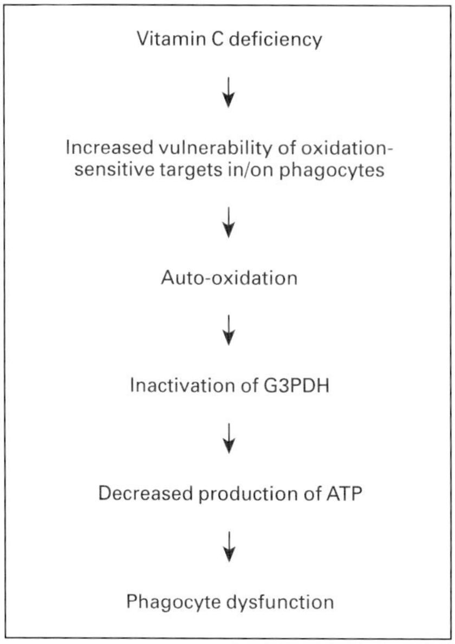

Fig. 1. Mechanism of abnormal phagocyte functions in vitamin C deficiency states.

glycolytic enzyme, glyceraldehyde-3-phosphate dehydrogenase (G3PDH), resulting in impairment of cellular energy metabolism and phagocyte dysfunction. Vitamin C protects G3PDH against HOCl-mediated oxidative inactivation during activation of phagocytes, and preserves the oxidation-sensitive functions of these cells [20]. This mechanism is summarized in figure 1.

Interestingly, vitamin C deficiency in humans is associated with anergy to various recall antigens, suggesting that this vitamin is also necessary for optimum activity of T lymphocytes [23]. There are at least two possible mechanisms by which this may be achieved. Firstly, although they do not produce significant amounts of reactive oxidants, the proliferative and cytokine-secreting functions of T lymphocytes are extremely sensitive to oxidative inactivation, particularly by HOCl [20, 24]. T lymphocytes operating in close proximity to activated phagocytes at sites of inflammatory reactions are therefore vulnerable, depending on the availability of vitamin C, to oxidant-mediated dysfunction [20].

Secondly, auto-oxidative inhibition of neutrophil chemotaxis as a consequence of hypovitaminosis C may result in a secondary decrease in the influx of $CD4^+$ T lymphocytes into sites of inflammation. Although speculative, this proposal is based on recent reports that neutrophil primary granules contain a series of well-characterized polypeptides (defensin-1, defensin-2 and CAP37/azurocidin) which are potent chemoattractants for $CD4^+$ T lymphocytes and

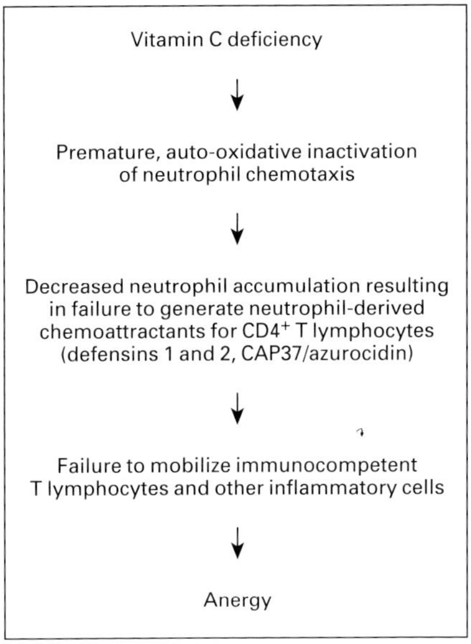

Fig. 2. Vitamin C and anergy.

macrophages [25, 26]. This may explain why neutrophil migration into sites of inflammation precedes, and may even be a prerequisite for the subsequent influx of T lymphocytes. Vitamin C deficiency may therefore lead to abnormal cell-mediated immune responses by compromising neutrophil chemotaxis and neutrophil-dependent recruitment of macrophages and T lymphocytes. These events are summarized in figure 2.

Anti-Inflammatory Properties of Vitamin C

As well as promoting optimum host defences, vitamin C may also restrict the wayward, pro-inflammatory and cytotoxic activities of the abundant, highly-aggressive, oxidant-generating phagocytic cells of the immune system. Although primarily antimicrobial, undiscerning phagocyte-derived reactive oxidants, when released extracellularly, present the potential hazard of oxidative damage and dysfunction to bystander host cells and tissues. If sustained, as is the case in cigarette smokers in whom there is chronic, smoke-mediated activation of circulating and pulmonary phagocytes, then accelerated development of degenerative disorders (pulmonary dysfunction and atherosclerosis) and inflammation-related epithelial cancers may ensue [27]. The spectrum of potentially harmful activities of phagocyte-derived reactive oxidants is

Table 2. Harmful activities of phagocyte-derived reactive oxidants

Activity	Mechanism
Cytotoxic for eukaryotic cells	Numerous, but interference with cellular energy metabolism may be particularly important
Pro-atherogenic	Oxidative modification of low-density lipoprotein
Pro-proteolytic	Oxidative inactivation of protease inhibitors, including α_1-antiprotease; oxidative activation of latent phagocyte-derived metalloproteases
Pro-adhesive	Upregulation of expression of adhesion molecules on vascular endothelium
Carcinogenic	Oxidative damage to DNA; inactivation of DNA repair enzymes
Immunosuppression	Oxidative inhibition of the functions of phagocytes, natural killer cells, B and T lymphocytes

shown in table 2. It is noteworthy that many of these are neutralized by vitamin C.

The relationship between phagocyte-derived oxidants and degenerative disorders and cancer is supported by consistent and compelling data from a number of large epidemiological studies which have demonstrated that the circulating leukocyte count, and the neutrophil count in particular, measured well before the development of manifest clinical disease are strong independent predictors of several cardiovascular conditions, including myocardial infarction, sudden cardiac death, all coronary heart disease combined, stroke and essential hypertension, as well as decline in pulmonary function (FEV_1), lung cancer incidence and mortality, possibly cancer at all sites and death from all causes [reviewed in 27]. It is noteworthy that the increments in circulating phagocyte counts which apparently predispose to degenerative diseases and cancer are relatively modest, being within the normal range for apparently healthy adults.

Interestingly, clinical disorders for which circulating leukocyte counts are predictive, are essentially the same as those which have been demonstrated in epidemiological studies to be associated with decreased dietary intake and/or plasma levels of antioxidative nutrients, including vitamin C. This is unlikely to be coincidental and suggests that the vitamin C requirements of an individual may be determined by the numbers and pro-oxidative activities of circulating phagocytes. This relationship is strengthened by an observed inverse relationship between the numbers and pro-oxidative activities of circulating neutrophils and plasma concentrations of vitamin C [28, 29].

Vitamin E and Host Defences

Administration of vitamin E to experimental animals and to young, healthy adult humans, as well as to elderly humans, is associated with increased mitogen-activated proliferation of circulating T lymphocytes and enhanced secretion of cytokines by unfractionated mononuclear leukocytes [24, 30]. These immunopotentiating effects of vitamin E have been attributed to an inhibitory effect of this agent on the production of the immunosuppressive prostaglandin, prostaglandin E_2, by these cells, as well as by macrophages [24, 30]. The mechanism by which vitamin E modulates production of prostaglandin E_2 has not been established, but may be related to inhibition of phospholipase A_2 (PLA_2) and/or cyclo-oxygenase [24, 30]. Since vitamin E has been reported to decrease the influx of Ca^{2+} into human epithelial cells [31], it is possible that this agent may regulate the Ca^{2+}-dependent activation of PLA_2 rather than its activity.

Neutralization of immunosuppressive lysophospholipids represents an alternative mechanism of vitamin E-mediated immunopotentiation. These polar lipids, which are generated as primary hydrolysis products during the cleavage of membrane phospholipids by PLA_2, possess potent detergent activity [32] and antimicrobial properties [33]. At concentrations which are within the range of those present in biological fluids [34], lysophosphatidylcholine (LPC) is directly cytotoxic for human lymphocytes, while at lower concentrations it is a potent inhibitor of Na^+, K^+-ATPase activity, the plasma membrane K^+-transporter of eukaryotic cells, which is indispensable for T lymphocyte proliferation [35]. Treatment of T lymphocytes with vitamin E not only abolishes the cytotoxic and antiproliferative Na^+, K^+-ATPase-inhibitory effects of exogenous LPC on these cells, but also neutralizes those of endogenously generated lysophospholipids following activation of PLA_2 [35, 36]. These cytoprotective, immunopotentiating effects of vitamin E are achieved by stabilizing the plasma membrane against the disruptive effects of lysophospholipids [32].

Anti-Inflammatory Properties of Vitamin E

As is the case with vitamin C, vitamin E possesses anti-inflammatory properties, providing a possible mechanistic basis for the data from epidemiological studies which have implicated this agent in the retardation or prevention of development of degenerative diseases and cancer. While the classical antioxidative properties of vitamin E are likely to contribute to the anti-inflammatory potential of this agent, other activities such as modulation of protein kinase C (PKC) in vascular smooth muscle cells [37], as well as neutralization of lysophospholipids are probably also involved. In the case of smooth muscle cells, binding of vitamin E to a putative receptor protein results in sequential activation of the cytosolic nuclear transcription factor, AP-1, and an uncharacterized protein phosphatase, which in turn causes dephosphorylative inactivation of PKC and inhibition of cellular proliferation [37]. This may be of importance in the prevention of ischaemic heart disease.

Notwithstanding their immunosuppressive properties, lysophospholipids are also potent pro-inflammatory agents, their spectrum of potentially harmful activities being remarkably similar to that of phagocyte-derived reactive oxidants. Lysophospholipids promote the adhesion of circulating leukocytes to vascular endothelium by upregulating the expression of the endothelial adhesion molecules, P-selectin and ICAM-1 [38]. They also cause enhanced production of reactive oxidants by phagocytes [39], and mast cell degranulation [40]. Some of these pro-inflammatory effects may be achieved by direct activation of PKC [41]. Alternatively, lysophospholipids may cause sublethal alterations in plasma membrane permeability to cations, resulting in uncontrolled influx of Ca^{2+} and hyperactivation of inflammatory cells [31, 42].

Lysophospholipids have been reported to be present in high concentrations in the bronchoalveolar lavage fluid of allergic subjects challenged with antigen, and may reach concentrations as high as 150 μM in the alveolar lining fluid in some individuals [34], and are thought to be involved in the aetiology of inflammation-related damage to the airways in asthmatic individuals [34, 43]. Lysophospholipids are also generated in large quantities by the heart during injury such as mycocardial ischaemia and probably contribute to the electrophysiologic alterations that lead to arrhythmogenesis [44]. In these settings, lysophospholipids may originate directly from inflammatory cells, or they may be formed as a result of the release of secretory PLA_2 by inflammatory cells such as mast cells and phagocytes [33, 43].

Vitamin E by virtue of its ability to neutralize lysophospholipids may therefore represent a first line of defence against these cytotoxic, pro-inflammatory agents. Investigations conducted in this laboratory [unpubl. data] have demonstrated that vitamin E protects a variety of cell types, including erythrocytes, ciliated respiratory epithelium, neutrophils and lymphocytes against the cytotoxic effects of LPC, and also inhibits the pro-inflammatory interactions of this lysophospholipid with human neutrophils in vitro.

Conclusions

Vitamins A, B_6, C, E and possibly D are necessary for efficient host defence against microbial and viral pathogens. The principle beneficiaries of optimum intake of these vitamins are likely to be infants and young children with immature, developing immune systems, and the elderly, many of whom have acquired, age-related immune dysfunction. Vitamins C and E also have anti-inflammatory properties, which, if operative in vivo, may explain their proposed roles in the risk reduction of degenerative diseases and cancer.

References

1 Sommer A: Vitamin A, infectious disease, and childhood mortality: A 2c solution? J Infect Dis 1993;167:1003–1007.

2 Semba RD, Miotti P, Chiphangwi JD, Henderson R, Dallabetaa G, Yang LP, Hoover D: Maternal vitamin A deficiency and child growth failure during human immunodeficiency virus infection. J Acquir Immune Defic Syndr Hum Retroviral 1997;14:219–222.

3 Coutsoudis A, Robat RA, Coovadia HM, Kuhn L, Tsai WY, Stein ZA: The effects of vitamin A supplementation on the morbidity of children born to HIV-infected women. Am J Publ Health 1995;85:1076–1081.

4 Coutsoudis A: The relationship between vitamin A status and immune function during measles. J Nutr Immunol 1995;1/2:111–132.

5 Benn CS, Aaby P, Balé C, Olsen J, Michaelsen K, George E: Randomised trial of effect of vitamin A supplementation on antibody response to measles vaccine in Guinea-Bissau, West Africa. Lancet 1997;350:101–105.

6 Semba R: Linking vitamin A and childhood immunizations. J Nutr Immunol 1995;1/2:87–109.

7 Smith SM, Hayes CE: Contrasting impairments in IgM and IgG responses of vitamin A-deficient mice. Proc Natl Acad Sci USA 1987;84:5878–5882.

8 Ross AC: Vitamin A status and the antibody response to bacterial antigens. J Nutr Immunol 1995; 1/2:47–75.

9 Cantorna MT, Nashold FE, Hayes CE: In vitamin A deficiency multiple mechanisms establish a regulatory T-helper cell imbalance with excess Th1 and insufficient Th2 function. J Immunol 1994; 152:1515–1522.

10 Santhi G, Ramanadham M: Intestinal mucosal immune response in experimental vitamin A deficiency: Reduction in helper T cell number and mitogenic stimulation of intestinal intraepithelial lymphocytes. J Nutr Immunol 1994;2:29–38.

11 Biesalski HK, Stofft E, Wellner U, Niederauer U, Bassler KH: Vitamin A and ciliated cells. I. Respiratory epithelia. Z Ernährungswiss 1986;25:114–122.

12 Meydani SN: Micronutrients and immune function in the elderly. Ann NY Acad Sci 1990;587: 196–207.

13 Miller LT, Kerkvliet NI: Effect of vitamin B_6 on immunocompetence in the elderly. Ann NY Acad Sci 1990;587:49–54.

14 Meydani SN, Ribaya-Mercado JD, Russel RM, Sayhoun N, Morrow FD, Gershoff SN: The effect of vitamin B_6 on the immune response of healthy elderly. Ann NY Acad Sci 1990;587:303–306.

15 Rook GW: The role of vitamin D in tuberculosis. Am Rev Respir Dis 1988;138:768–770.

16 Studzinski GP, Moore DC: Sunlight – Can it prevent as well as cause cancer? Cancer Res 1995; 55:4014–4022.

17 Warwick-Davies J, Dhillon J, O'Brien L, Andrew PW, Lowrie DB: Apparent killing of *Mycobacterium tuberculosis* by cytokine-activated human monocytes can be an artefact of a cytotoxic effect on the monocytes. Clin Exp Immunol 1994;96:214–217.

18 Kawa S, Nikaido T, Aoki Y, Zhai Y, Kumagai T, Furihata K, Fuji S, Kiyosawa K: Vitamin D analogues up-regulate p21 and p27 during growth inhibition of pancreatic cancer cell lines. Br J Can 1997;76:884–886.
19 Young MRI, Halpin J, Wang J, Wright MA, Matthews J, Pak AS: 1α,25-Dihydroxyvitamin D_3 plus γ-interferon blocks lung tumour production of granulocyte-macrophage colony-stimulating factor and induction of immunosuppressor cells. Cancer Res 1993;53:6006–6010.
20 Anderson R, Smit MJ, Jooné GK, Van Staden AM: Vitamin C and cellular immune functions: Protection against hypochlorous acid-mediated inactivation of glyceraldehyde-3-phosphate dehydrogenase and ATP generation in human leukocytes as a possible mechanism of ascorbate-mediated immunostimulation. Ann NY Acad Sci 1990;587:34–48.
21 Hunt C, Chakravorty NK, Annan G, Habibzadeh N, Schorah CJ: The clinical effects of vitamin C supplementation in elderly hospitalised patients with acute respiratory infections. Int J Vitam Nutr Res 1994;64:212–219.
22 Levy R, Shriker O, Porath A, Riesenberg K, Schlaeffer F: Vitamin C for the treatment of recurrent furunculosis in patients with impaired neutrophil functions. J Infect Dis 1996;173:1502–1505.
23 Jacob RA, Kelley DS, Pianalto FS, Swendseid ME, Hennig SM, Zhang JZ, Ames BW, Fraga CJ, Peters JH: Immunocompetence and oxidant defense during ascorbate depletion of healthy men. Am J Clin Nutr 1991;54(suppl):1302–1309.
24 Jeng KCG, Yang CS, Siu WY, Tsai YS, Liao WJ, Kuo JS: Supplementation with vitamins C and E enhances cytokine production by peripheral blood mononuclear cells in healthy adults. Am J Clin Nutr 1996;64:960–965.
25 Taub DD, Anver M, Oppenheim JJ, Longo DL, Murphy WJ: T lymphocyte recruitment by interleukin-8 (IL-8): IL-8-induced degranulation of neutrophils releases potent chemoattractants for human T lymphocytes both in vitro and in vivo. J Clin Invest 1996;97:1931–1941.
26 Chertov O, Michiel DF, Xu L, Ming Wong J, Tani K, Murphy WJ, Longo DL, Taub DD, Oppenheim JJ: Identification of defensin-1, defensin-2, and CAP37/azurocidin as T-cell chemoattractant proteins released from interleukin-8-stimulated neutrophils. J Biol Chem 1996;271:2935–2940.
27 Anderson R, Van Antwerpen VL: Vitamins in the maintenance of optimum immune functions and in the prevention of phagocyte-mediated tissue damage and carcinogenesis; in Walter P (ed): The Scientific Basis for Vitamin Intake in Human Nutrition. Bibl Nutr Dieta. Basel, Karger, 1995, vol 52, pp 66–74.
28 Van Antwerpen VL, Theron AJ, Myer MS, Richards GA, Wolmarans L, Booysen U, Van der Merwe CA, Sluis-Cremer GK, Anderson R: Cigarette smoke-mediated oxidant stress, phagocytes, vitamin C, vitamin E, and tissue injury. Ann NY Acad Sci 1993;686:53–65.
29 Winklhofer-Roob BM, Ellemunter H, Frühwirth M, Schlegel-Haueter SE, Khoschsorur G, van't Hof MA, Shmerling DH: Plasma vitamin C concentrations in patients with cystic fibrosis: Evidence of associations with lung inflammation. Am J Clin Nutr 1997;65:1858–1866.
30 Meydani SN, Wu D, Santos MS, Hayek MG: Antioxidant and immune responses in aged persons: Overview of present evidence. Am J Clin Nutr 1995;62(suppl):1462–1476.
31 Goswami SK, Marom Z: Vitamin E-induced inhibition of mucin secretion in an epithelial cell line: Involvement of calcium. Am J Respir Crit Care Med 1997;155:A433.
32 Kagan VE: Tocopherol stabilizes membrane against phospholipase A, free fatty acids and lysophospholipids. Ann NY Acad Sci 1989;570:121–135.
33 Van Rensburg CEJ, Jooné GK, O'Sullivan JF, Anderson R: Antimicrobial activities of clofazimine and B669 are mediated by lysophospholipids. Antimicrob Agents Chemother 1992;36:2729–2735.
34 Chilton FH, Averill FJ, Hubbard WC, Fonteh AN, Triggiani M, Liu MC: Antigen-induced generation of lyso-phospholipids in human airways. J Exp Med 1996;183:2235–2245.
35 Anderson R, Smit MJ, Van Rensburg CEJ: Lysophospholipid-mediated inhibition of Na^+, K^+-adenosine triphosphatase is a possible mechanism of immunosuppressive activity of cyclosporin A. Mol Pharmacol 1994;44:605–614.
36 Anderson R, Smit MJ: Clofazimine and B669 inhibit the proliferative responses and Na^+, K^+-adenosine triphosphatase activity of human lymphocytes by a lysophospholipid-dependent mechanism. Biochem Pharmacol 1993;46:2029–2038.

37 Azzi A, Boscoboinik D, Marilley D, Özer NK, Stäuble B, Tasinato A: Vitamin E: A sensor and an information transducer of the cell oxidation state. Am J Clin Nutr 1995;62(suppl):1337–1346.
38 Scalia R, Murohara T, Campbell B, Kaji A, Lefer AM: Lysophosphatidylcholine stimulates leukocyte rolling and adherence in rat mesenteric microvasculature. Am J Physiol 1997;272:H2584–H2590.
39 Ginsburg I, Ward PA, Varani J: Lysophosphatides enhance superoxide responses of stimulated human neutrophils. Inflammation 1989;13:163–174.
40 Marquardt DL, Walker LL: Lysophosphatidylcholine induces mast cell secretion and protein kinase C activation. J Allergy Clin Immunol 1991;88:721–730.
41 Oishi K, Ranor RL, Charp PA, Kuo JF: Regulation of protein kinase C by lysophospholipids: Potential role in signal transduction. J Biol Chem 1988;263:6865–6871.
42 Woodley SL, Ikenouchi H, Barry WH: Lysophosphatidylcholine increases cytosolic calcium in ventricular myocytes by direct action on the sacrolemma. J Moll Cell Cardiol 1991;23:671–680.
43 Mehta D, Gupta S, Gaur SN, Gangal SV, Agrawal KP: Increased leukocyte phospholipase A_2 activity and plasma lysophosphatidylcholine levels in asthma and rhinitis and their relationship to airway sensitivity to histamine. Am Rev Respir Dis 1990;142:157–161.
44 Man RY: Lysophosphatidylcholine-induced arrhythmias and its accumulation in the rat perfused heart. Br J Pharmacol 1998;93:412–416.

Prof. R. Anderson, University of Pretoria, Department of Immunology,
Medical Research Council Unit for Inflammation & Immunity,
PO Box 2034, Pretoria 0001, ZA (South Africa)
Tel. +27 12 319 2425, Fax +27 12 323 0732, E-Mail randerso@postillion.up.ac.za

Walter P, Hornig D, Moser U (eds): Functions of Vitamins beyond Recommended Dietary Allowances. Bibl Nutr Dieta. Basel, Karger, 2001, No 55, pp 148–158

Vitamin E and Immune Response in the Aged

Simin Nikbin Meydani, Alison A. Beharka

Nutritional Immunology Laboratory, Jean Mayer USDA Human Nutrition Research Center on Aging at Tufts University, Boston, Mass., USA

Vitamin E is the most effective chain-breaking, lipid-soluble antioxidant in biologic membranes of all cells, but it is found in especially high concentrations in the membranes of immune cells because their high polyunsaturated fatty acid content puts them at especially high risk for oxidative damage [Coquette et al., 1986; Hatman and Kayden, 1979]. Free radical damage to immune cell membrane lipids may ultimately impair the ability of immune cells to respond normally to challenge. Several animal and human studies have shown that vitamin E deficiency is associated with an inadequate immune response, whereas higher than recommended amounts have, in some instances, improved immunity. Vitamin E, long recognized as an essential nutrient for humans and animals, has recently been implicated in the reduction of risk for several immune and inflammatory diseases associated with aging.

Vitamin E and the Aging Immune Response

Laboratory Animals

The aging process is associated with depression of the immune system, and this decline in immunologic vigor contributes to the increased vulnerability of older individuals to infections and neoplastic disease compared with their young counterparts. This documented depression in immunity with age is due at least in part to an increase in the free radical burden associated with aging. Therefore, the level of dietary antioxidants, such as vitamin E, needed for normal immune function in the elderly may be higher than the current RDA.

This hypothesis, although not universally held, is supported by a growing body of research.

Vitamin E supplementation has been successfully used to improve some aspects of the age-related decline in laboratory animal immune function [Harman, 1980]. Meydani et al. [1986b] showed that increasing the level of dietary vitamin E from 30 to 500 ppm significantly increases delayed-type hypersensitivity (DTH) skin response, lymphocyte proliferation to Concanavalin A (Con A), and interleukin (IL)-2 production in old mice; this effect of vitamin E was associated with a decrease in prostaglandin (PG) E_2 production. Vitamin E-supplemented animals from this study also had a lower incidence of kidney amyloidosis than control (30 ppm vitamin E) animals [Meydani et al., 1986a]. In another study, Meydani et al. [1988] showed that while vitamin E supplementation did not have an effect on natural killer cell (NK) activity of unchallenged young or old mice, it was effective in preventing SRBC-induced suppression of NK activity in old mice.

Human Studies

Vitamin E supplementation has been shown to enhance immunity in elderly populations. Ziemlanski et al. [1986] supplemented institutionalized healthy elderly women with 100 mg vitamin E twice daily and assessed serum proteins and immunoglobulin concentrations after 4 and 12 months. Vitamin E increased total serum protein with the principal effect seen in the α_2- and β_2-globulin fractions occurring at 4 months. No significant effects were noted in the levels of either immunoglobulins or complement C3 after 12 months, although there was a significant increase in serum protein concentration. However, in another group, vitamin C along with vitamin E displayed significant increases in IgG and complement C3 levels.

Harman and Miller [1986] supplemented 103 elderly patients from a chronic care facility with 200 or 400 mg daily α-tocopherol acetate but did not see any beneficial effect on antibody development against influenza virus vaccine. Unfortunately, data on the subjects' health status, medication use, antibody levels, and other relevant parameters were not reported.

In a double-blind, placebo-controlled study, Meydani et al. [1990a] supplemented 34 healthy men and women (>60 years of age) with either a soybean oil placebo or 800 mg dl-α-tocopherol (400 mg capsules twice daily) for 30 days. The study evaluated the subjects' DTH, mitogenic response, and IL-1, IL-2, and PGE_2 production. Vitamin E supplementation was associated with increases in plasma vitamin E, DTH score, mitogenic response to Con A, and IL-2 production. Vitamin E supplementation was associated with decreases in PHA-stimulated PGE_2 production by peripheral blood mononuclear cells (PBMC) as well as plasma lipid peroxide levels. IL-1 production and PHAinduced proliferation of PBMC were not affected by vitamin E supplementation.

In a recent study, Meydani et al. [1997] supplemented healthy elderly (>65 years old) with placebo, 60, 200 or 800 mg/day of dl-α-tocopherol for 235 days using a double-blind, randomized design. All three vitamin E doses significantly enhanced DTH. Subjects consuming 200 mg/day vitamin E had the highest percent increase in DTH. The median percent change in DTH in the subjects supplemented with 200 mg/day vitamin E (65%) was significantly higher than that of the placebo group (17%). Although the median percent change in the groups supplemented with 60 and 800 mg/day vitamin E (41 and 49%, respectively) were similar to the 65% change observed in the 200-mg/day group, these changes did not reach statistical significance compared with those of the placebo group. There was no significant effect of supplementation with 60 mg/day in response to hepatitis B or tetanus and diphtheria vaccines. However, a significant increase in antibody response to hepatitis B was observed in subjects consuming 200 or 800 mg/day. Those consuming 200 mg/day also had a significant increase in antibody response to tetanus toxoid vaccine. There was no effect of vitamin E supplementation on the level of two autoantibodies, anti-DNA and antithyroglobulin, or the ability of neutrophils to kill *Candida albicans*. These data suggest that while supplementation with 60 mg/day vitamin E might enhance DTH, it is not adequate to cause a significant increase in antibody titer against hepatitis B or tetanus toxoid. Supplementation with 200 mg/day vitamin E, however, caused a significant increase in DTH and antibody response, and the magnitude of response for both indices was higher than those observed in the two other vitamin E groups. Thus, it was concluded that 200 mg/day represents the optimal level of vitamin E for the immune response of the elderly. The observation that the optimal response was detected in the 200 mg/day group suggests that there may be a threshold level for the immunostimulatory effect of vitamin E. Interestingly, vitamin E-supplemented subjects had 30% lower incidence of self-reported infections indicating that the immunostimulatory effect of vitamin E might have clinical significance for the elderly.

No adverse effects on the immune indices tested due to short-term, high-dose vitamin E supplementation were observed. Recently, the safety of 4 months of supplementation with 60, 200 and 800 IU/day of dl-α-tocopherol on general health, nutrient status, liver enzyme function, thyroid hormones, creatinine levels, serum autoantibodies, killing of *C. albicans* by neutrophils, and bleeding time in elderly subjects was assessed. Supplementation with vitamin E at these levels and for this period of time had no adverse effects on these parameters [Meydani et al., 1998]. Other studies are needed to determine the possible adverse effects of supplementation with larger doses of vitamin E for longer periods of time.

In another study, Cannon et al. [1990] supplemented young (22–29 years) and old (55–74 years) subjects with 400 IU dl-α-tocopherol twice daily for 48 days before undergoing eccentric exercise (downhill running). They reported that young subjects consuming placebo capsules had a significantly greater neutrophilia and plasma creatine kinase in response to eccentric exercise compared with old subjects consuming placebo. Vitamin E supplementation eliminated the age difference in neutrophilia and creatine kinase. In a subsequent report, Cannon et al. [1991] demonstrated that although vitamin E supplementation did not affect production of IL-1 or TNF, it prevented the eccentric exercise-induced rise in IL-1. Vitamin E supplementation, however, inhibited the production of another cytokine, IL-6. Since IL-1 and IL-6 have been implicated in the inflammatory process and the acute phase response and IL-1 has been found to be involved in exercise-induced muscle proteolysis and damage, their inhibition by vitamin E during damaging exercise could have practical implications. These studies indicated that in addition to its enhancement of cell-mediated immunity, vitamin E, by its modulation of cytokine production, can affect the catabolic consequences of the inflammatory process and acute phase response.

Several epidemiologic studies have investigated the interaction between vitamin E supplementation and immune function of free living elderly. Goodwin and Garry [1983] studied a population of healthy adults (65–94 years old) consuming high doses of vitamin E and did not find any correlation between vitamin E intake and DTH, mitogen-stimulated lymphocyte proliferation, serum antibodies, or circulating immune complexes. In this study, subjects taking supplemental doses of vitamin E greater than 5 times the RDA had lower absolute circulating lymphocyte counts than the rest of the population. Unfortunately, the results from this study are confounded by the fact that the subjects were consuming high doses of several vitamin supplements in addition to vitamin E.

Chavance et al. [1984, 1985] conducted a community-based survey on the relationship between nutritional and immunologic status in 100 healthy subjects over 60 years of age. They reported that plasma vitamin E levels were positively correlated with positive DTH responses to diphtheria toxoid, *C. albicans*, and trichophyton. In men only, positive correlations were also observed between vitamin E levels and the number of positive DTH responses. Subjects with tocopherol levels >135 mg/l were found to have higher helper-inducer/cytotoxic-suppressor ratios. Blood vitamin E concentrations were also negatively correlated with the number of infectious disease episodes in the preceding year.

Payette et al. [1990] reported a negative correlation between dietary vitamin E and ex vivo IL-2 production in free-living elderly Canadians. This result is suspect, however, because 70% of the presumably 'healthy' elderly in this study had undetectable IL-2 levels. Others have reported that while IL-2 production in healthy older adults is about one-half to two-thirds that of young subjects, it is still detectable [Meydani et al., 1990a, b, Nagel et al. 1988]. The study is further complicated because dietary vitamin E intake rather than plasma vitamin E level was used as the indicator of a subject's tocopherol status. Nutrient databases for vitamin E are incomplete and do not necessarily represent the actual tocopherol status of a given individual.

Clinical Implications of the Immunostimulating Effect of Vitamin E

The immunostimulatory effect of vitamin E has been shown to be associated with increased resistance to infectious diseases. Tengerdy et al. [1978] showed that supplementation with 150–300 mg/kg vitamin E significantly reduced *Escherichia coli*-induced mortality in chickens (from 50 to 5%). Similarly, the mortality of mice infected with Diplococcus pneumonia type I decreased from 80 to 20% after vitamin E supplementation [Heinzerling et al., 1974]. The protective effect of vitamin E was associated with higher antibody titer, increased plaque-forming units, and higher phagocytic activity. Colnago et al. [1984] showed that supplementation with vitamin E decreased mortality in chickens infected with *Eimeria tenella* (coccidiosis). Decreased mortality and lesion scores from *Histomonas melacardis* infection were also reported in turkeys supplemented with 500 IU/kg vitamin E [Schildknecht and Squibb, 1979]. Vitamin E-deficient pigs [Teige et al., 1978] had higher mortality and more pronounced clinical pathology from experimentally-induced swine dysentery than those receiving adequate levels of vitamin E. Furthermore, vitamin E supplementation in pigs was shown to increase resistance against *E. coli* [Ellis and Vorhies, 1986] and *Treponema hydysenteriae* [Teige et al., 1982]. Increased resistance to chlamydia in sheep and lambs by vitamin E was also reported [Stephens et al., 1979, Nockels, 1979]. Reddy et al. [1985] reported that serum from vitamin E-supplemented calves inhibited proliferation of rhinotracheitis virus more effectively than serum from control calves.

The potential benefits of dietary supplementation of vitamin E in HIV infection and AIDS has been investigated in mice infected with a murine leukemia retrovirus. Vitamin E supplementation decreased retrovirus-induced T-cell suppressor activity and increased IL-2 production. The researchers concluded that vitamin E may reverse certain immunosuppressive effects of retroviral infection [Kline et al., 1990]. Vitamin E supplementation also decreased indices of lipid peroxidation and decreased the size and frequency of induced esophageal tumors in retrovirus-infected mice and nonimmunocompromised mice [Odeleye et al., 1992]. In another study of retrovirus-infected mice, vitamin E supplementation significantly restored T- and B-cell proliferation and stimulated NK activity, which had been suppressed by retroviral infection. These researchers concluded that vitamin E can help to normalize retrovirus-induced immune defects during progression of murine AIDS and suggested that vitamin E could be a potential therapeutic co-nutrient to modify human immune dysfunction caused by HIV infection [Wang et al., 1994]. Studies to determine clinical benefits of vitamin E supplementation in animal models of HIV infection or in HIV-infected humans are needed before the preventive and/or therapeutic potential of vitamin E can be determined.

Hayek et al. [1997b] fed young and old mice either 30 or 500 ppm vitamin E for 8 weeks, at which time they were infected with influenza virus. Old mice fed 30 ppm of vitamin E had higher viral titer than young mice fed 30 ppm vitamin E. Influenza lung viral titers were lower in old mice fed 500 ppm vitamin E compared with the age-matched mice fed 30 ppm vitamin E. The authors suggested that the effect of vitamin E may be due, in part, to preservation of antioxidant status and NK cell activity because old mice fed 500 ppm vitamin E maintained a higher antioxidant index than age-matched controls and the age-associated decline in NK activity was prevented by feeding old infected mice 500 ppm vitamin E. Furthermore, vitamin E supplementation at 500 ppm did not affect secondary splenic cytotoxic T-cell activity or primary pulmonary CTL activity in this study. However, the mechanism for the effect of vitamin E on reducing influenza viral titer is still unclear.

Mechanisms of Vitamin E Effect

The mechanism behind the immunostimulatory effect of vitamin E has eluded scientists to this day. However, there is compelling evidence suggesting that vitamin E exerts its immunoenhancing effect by either reducing prostaglandin synthesis [Meydani et al., 1986b, 1990a] and/or decreasing free radical formation [Corwin and Schloss, 1980].

Increased free radical formation, whether due to aging, environmental pollutants or diet, damages the components of the immune system. Oxygen metabolites, especially H_2O_2, produced by activated macrophages depress lymphocyte proliferation [Metzger et al., 1980]. Tocopherol has been shown to decrease H_2O_2 formation by PMN [Baehner et al., 1977]. Additionally, the immunosuppressive effect of vitamin E deficiency appears to be due to increased free radical reactions that result in increased nonenzyme-catalyzed lipid peroxidation as well as enzyme-catalyzed lipid peroxidation, i.e. formation of PGE_2. Macrophages from vitamin E-deficient rats showed a 3-fold increase in chemiluminescence and increase in membrane viscosity compared with those from control rats [Sharmanov et al., 1986]. Harris et al. [1980] also showed increased O_2 consumption and H_2O_2 release in rats fed vitamin E-deficient diets. Neutrophils from vitamin E-deficient rats had more peroxidized lipids in their membranes, produced more H_2O_2, and exhibited lower phagocytosis and chemotaxis than vitamin E-supplemented rats [Machlin, 1991].

Increased production of lipid peroxides caused by vitamin E deficiency can affect the physical properties of cellular and subcellular organelles crucial for the normal function of the immune cells. This notion is supported by the observation that vitamin E deficiency in rats decreased the membrane fluidity of platelets [Carpenter, 1986]. Furthermore, electron micrographs of lymphocyte mitochondrial membrane from vitamin E-deficient rats showed swollen and disrupted areas [Lehman and McGill, 1986].

Vitamin E supplementation may provide protection for the cells of the immune system against oxidative damage. Villa et al. [1986] reported that vitamin E supplementation in vitro caused a concentration-dependent inhibition of arachidonic acid-induced aggregation of PMN and mononuclear leukocytes. They suggested that this may have been due to interference with lipoxygenase activity. Topika et al. [1989] found that the addition of α-tocopherol (0.2 μmol/l) to human lymphocytes in vitro suppressed lipid peroxidation and oxidant damage to DNA when induced by the catalytic system of Fe^{2+}-sodium ascorbate. Sepe and Clark [1985] studied neutrophil lysis in liposome target vesicles, demonstrating that stimulated neutrophils secrete myeloperoxidase and H_2O_2, which combine with extracellular lipids to form a membrane lytic system. In vitro addition of α-tocopherol to the liposomes increased their resistance to the myeloperoxidase-H_2O_2 system.

In addition to its reduction of nonenzymatic products of lipid peroxidation, vitamin E may also modulate immune responsiveness through its effect on the synthesis of arachidonic acid metabolites. At low concentrations, PGE_2 is believed to be necessary for certain aspects of cellular immunity; however, at higher concentrations, PGE_2 has a suppressive effect on several indices of cellular and humoral immunity, such as antibody formation, DTH, lymphocyte proliferation and cytokine production. Vitamin E deficiency was shown to increase the production of eicosanoids, while vitamin E supplementation decreased their formation [Meydani et al., 1986b]. Beharka et al. [1997] used an in vitro co-culture system in which purified macrophages and T cells from young and old mice were cultured together to demonstrate that macrophages from old mice were inhibitory to T cells from young mice due, at least in part, to increased macrophage production of PGE_2. Vitamin E improved T-cell responsiveness in this system by reducing macrophage PGE_2 production, although a direct effect of vitamin E on T cells was also observed. Furthermore, Wu et al. [1996] demonstrated that vitamin E supplementation of old mice decreased the age-associated increase in PGE_2 production and inducible cyclooxygenase (COX)-2 activity in macrophages from old mice [Hayek et al., 1997a]. Further studies are needed to determine the direct effect of vitamin E on T cells and its contribution to the immunostimulatory effect of vitamin E. Thus, it appears that vitamin E enhancement of the aged immune system is mostly mediated through a decrease in PGE_2 production.

Conclusion

It is indisputable that adequate vitamin E is essential for normal immune function. Vitamin E deficiency impairs several aspects of the immune response, including B- and T-cell-mediated immunity as well as the function of phagocytic cells. However, the level of vitamin E needed to alleviate deficiency does not appear to be the optimal level needed for ideal immune function under all conditions. Supplementation with higher than recommended levels of vitamin E has been shown to enhance the immune responsiveness of older adults and animal. This effect is more pronounced when free radical formation and lipid peroxidation are increased due to exposure to environmental pollutants, consumption of high dietary polyunsaturated acids, and aging. Because several animal studies have shown increased resistance to bacterial and viral diseases with vitamin E supplementation, the increase in immune response due to vitamin E supplementation is of clinical significance.

Therefore, the immunostimulatory effect of vitamin E warrants further well-controlled, long-term human studies to determine the appropriate level of vitamin E for optimal function of the immune response in humans of different ages. Such studies should include clinically relevant indices of the immune system. Carefully designed clinical trials and epidemiologic studies are also needed to determine the clinical relevance of vitamin E-induced immunostimulation, i.e. its impact on immune-related diseases. More importantly, the mechanism of the immunoregulatory effect of vitamin E needs to be further delineated if its immunoenhancing properties are to be fully utilized.

Acknowledgments

The authors' work has been funded at least in part with Federal funds from the US Department of Agriculture, Agricultural Research Service under contract No. 53-K06-01, NIA Grant No. AG09140, USDA Grant No. 94-37200-0489, and Roche Vitamins, Inc. The contents of this publication do not necessarily reflect the views or policies of the US Department of Agriculture, nor does mention of trade names, commercial products, or organizations imply endorsement by the US Government. The authors thank Timothy S. McElreavy, MA, for preparation of the manuscript.

References

Baehner RL, Boxer LA, Allen JM, et al: Autooxidation as a basis for altered function by polymorphonuclear leukocytes. Blood 1977;50:327–35.

Beharka AA, Wu D, Han SN, et al: Macrophage prostaglandin production contributes to the age-associated decrease in T cell function which is reversed by the dietary antioxidant vitamin E. Mech Ageing Dev 1997;93:59–77.

Cannon JG, Orencole SF, Fielding RA, et al: Acute phase response in exercise: Interaction of age and vitamin E on neutrophils and muscle enzyme release. Am J Physiol 1990;259:R1214–R1219.

Cannon JG, Meydani SN, Fielding RA, et al: Acute phase response in exercise. II. Associations between vitamin E, cytokines, and muscle proteolysis. Am J Physiol 1991;260:R1235–R1240.

Carpenter MP: Effects of vitamin E on the immune system; in Meyskens FL, Prasad KN (eds): Vitamins and Cancer. Basel, Karger, 1986, pp 199–211.

Chavance M, Brubacher G, Herbeth B, et al: Immunological and nutritional status among the elderly; in De Wick AL (ed): Lymphoid Cell Functions in Aging. Interlaken, Eurage, 1984, pp 231–237.

Chavance M, Brubacher G, Herbert B, et al: Immunological nutritional status among the elderly; in Chandra RK (ed): Nutritional Immunity and Illness in the Elderly. New York, Pergamon Press, 1985, pp 137–142.

Colnago GL, Jensen LS, Long PL: Effect of selenium and vitamin E on the development of immunity to coccidiosis in chickens. Poult Sci 1984;63:1136–1143.

Coquette A, Vray B, Vanderpas J: Role of vitamin E in the protection of the resident macrophage membrane against oxidative damage. Arch Int Physiol Biochem 1986;94:529–534.

Corwin LM, Schloss J: Role of antioxidants on the stimulation of the mitogen response. J Nutr 1980; 110:2497–2505.

Ellis RP, Vorhies MW: Effect of supplemental dietary vitamin E on the serologic response of swine to an *Escherichia coli* bacterium. J Am Vet Med Assoc 1986;168:231–232.

Goodwin JS, Garry TJ: Relationship between megadoses vitamin supplementation and immunological function in a healthy elderly polulation. Clin Exp Immunol 1983;51:647–653.

Harman D: Free radical theory of aging: Beneficial effect of antioxidants on the lifespan of male NZB mice; role of free radical reactions in the deterioration of the immune system with age and in the pathogenesis of systemic lupus erythematosus. Age 1980;3:64–73.

Harman D, Miller RW: Effect of vitamin E on the immune response to influenza virus vaccine and the incidence of infectious disease in man. Age 1986;9:21–23.

Harris RE, Boxer LA, Baehner RL: Consequences of vitamin E deficiency on the phagocyte and oxidative function of the rat polymorphonuclear leukocyte. Blood 1980;55:338–343.

Hatman LJ, Kayden HJ: A high-performance liquid chromatographic method for the determination of tocopherol in plasma and cellular elements of the blood. J Lipid Res 1979;20:639–645.

Hayek MG, Mura CV, Wu D, et al: Enhanced expression of inducible cyclooxygenase with age in murine macrophages. J Immunol 1997a;159:2445–2451.

Hayek MG, Taylor SF, Bender BS, et al: Vitamin E supplementation decreases lung viral titer in mice infected with influenza. J Infect Dis 1997b;176:273–276.

Heinzerling RH, Tengerdy RP, Wick LL, et al: Vitamin E protects mice against Diplococcus pneumonia type I infection. Infect Immun 1974;10:1292–1295.
Kline K, Rao A, Romach E, et al: Vitamin E effects on retrovirus-induced immune dysfunctions. Ann NY Acad Sci 1990;587:294–296.
Lehman J, McGill M: Biomedical and ultrastructural alterations in platelets, reticulocytes and lymphocytes from rats fed vitamin E-deficient diets. J Lipid Res 1986;23:299–306.
Machlin LJ: Vitamin E; in Machlin LJ (ed): Handbook of Vitamins: Nutritional, Biochemical, and Clinical Aspects, ed 2. New York, Dekker, 1991, pp 99–144.
Metzger Z, Hoffeld JT, Oppenheim JJ: Macrophage-mediated suppression. I. Evidence for participation of both hydrogen peroxide and prostaglandin of suppression of murine lymphocyte proliferation. J Immunol 1980;124:983–988.
Meydani SN, Cathcart ES, Hopkins RE, et al: Antioxidants in experimental amyloidosis of young and old mice; in Glenner GG, Asserman EP, Benditt E, et al (eds): Fourth International Symposium on Amyloidosis. New York, Plenum Press, 1986a, pp 683–692.
Meydani SN, Meydani M, Verdon CP, et al: Vitamin E supplementation suppresses prostaglandin E_2 synthesis and enhances the immune response of aged mice. Mech Age Dev 1986b;34:191–201.
Meydani SN, Stocking LM, Shapiro AC, et al: Fish oil- and tocopherol-induced changes in ex vivo synthesis of spleen and lung leukotriene B_4 in mice. Ann NY Acad Sci 1988;524:395–397.
Meydani SN, Barklund MP, Liu S, et al: Vitamin E supplementation enhances cell-mediated immunity in healthy elderly subjects. Am J Clin Nutr 1990a;52:557–563.
Meydani SN, Meydani M, Blumberg JB: Antioxidants and the aging immune response. Adv Exp Med Biol 1990b;262:57–68.
Meydani SN, Meydani M, Blumberg JB, et al: Vitamin E supplementation enhances in vivo immune response in healthy elderly: A dose-response study. JAMA 1997;277:1380–1386.
Meydani SN, Meydani M, Blumberg JB, et al: Assessment of the safety of supplementation with different levels of vitamin E in healthy older adults. Am J Clin Nutr 1998;68:311–318.
Nagel JE, Chorpa RK, Chrest FJ, et al: Decreased proliferation, interleukin-2 synthesis, and interleukin-2 receptor expression are accompanied by decreased mRNA expression in phytohemagglutin-stimulated cells from elderly donors. J Clin Invest 1988;81:1096–1102.
Nockels CF: Protective Effects of supplemental vitamin E against infection. Fed Proc 1979;38:2134–2138.
Odeleye OE, Eskelson CD, Mufti SI, et al: Vitamin E protection against nitrosamine-induced esophageal tumor incidence in mice immunocompromised by retroviral infection. Carcinogenesis 1992;13: 1811–1816.
Payette H, Rola-Pleszczynski M, Ghadririan P: Nutritional factors in relation to cellular and regulatory immune variables in free-living elderly population. Am J Clin Nutr 1990;33:606–608.
Reddy PG, Morrill JL, Minocha HC, et al: Effects of supplemental vitamin E on the immune system of calves. J Dairy Sci 1985;69:164–171.
Schildknecht EG, Squibb RL: The effect of vitamins A, E, and K on experimentally induced histomoniasis in turkeys. Parisitology 1979;78:19–31.
Sepe SM, Clark RA: Oxidant membrane injury by the neutrophil myeloperoxidase system. II. Injury by stimulated neutrophils and protection by lipid-soluble antioxidants. J Immunol 1985;134:1896–1901.
Sharmanov AT, Aidarkhanov BB, Kurmangaliev SM: Effect of vitamin E on oxidative metabolism of macrophages. Bull Exp Biol Med 1986;101:723–725.
Stephens LC, McChesney AE, Nockels CF: Improved recovery of vitamin-E-treated lambs that have been experimentally infected with intratracheal Chlamydia. Br Vet J 1979;135:291–293.
Teige J, Saxegaard F, Frooslie A: Influence of diet on experimental swine dysentery. 2. Effects of a vitamin E- and selenium-deficient diet supplemented with 3% cod liver oil, vitamin E, or selenium. Acta Vet Scand 1978;19:133–146.
Teige J, Tollersrud S, Lund A, et al: Swine dysentery: The influence of dietary vitamin E and selenium on the clinical and pathological effect of *Treponema hyodysenteriae* infection in pigs. Res Vet Sci 1982;32:95–160.
Tengerdy RP, Heinzerling RH, Mathias MM: Effect of vitamin E on disease resistance and immune response; in de Dune C, Hayaishi O (eds): Tocopherol, Oxygen and Biomembranes. New York, Elsevier, 1978, pp 191–200.

Topika J, Binkovaa B, Sram RJ, et al: The influence of alpha-tocopherol and pyritinol on oxidative DNA damage and lipid peroxidation in human lymphocytes. Mutat Res 1989;225:131–136.
Villa S, Lorico A, Morazzoni G, et al: Vitamin E and vitamin C inhibits arachidonic-induced aggregation of human peripheral blood leukocyte in vitro. Agents Actions 1986;19:127–131.
Wang Y, Huang DS, Eskelson CD, et al: Long-term dietary vitamin E retards development of retrovirus-induced dysregulation in cytokine production. Clin Immunol Immunopathol 1994;72:70–75.
Wu D, Han SN, Meydani SN: Vitamin E supplementation inhibits macrophage cyclooxygenase activity of old mice. FASEB J 1996;9:A191.
Ziemlanski S, Wartanowicz M, Klos A, et al: The effect of ascorbic acid and alpha-tocopherol supplementation on serum proteins and immunoglobulin concentration in the elderly. Nutr Int 1986;2:1–5.

Prof. S.N. Meydani, Tufts University, USDA Human Nutrition, Research Center on Aging,
711 Washington Street, Boston MA 02111-1524 (USA)
Tel. +1 617 556 3129, Fax +1 617 556 3344, E-Mail s_meeydani_im@hnrc.tufts.edu

Walter P, Hornig D, Moser U (eds): Functions of Vitamins beyond Recommended Dietary Allowances. Bibl Nutr Dieta. Basel, Karger, 2001, No 55, pp 159–170

Vitamin K and Tissue Mineralization

Cees Vermeer [a], *Henk H.W. Thijssen* [b], *Karly Hamulyák* [c]

Departments of [a] Biochemistry and [b] Pharmacology, Maastricht University and [c] Department of Hematology, University Hospital, Maastricht, The Netherlands

Vitamin K is a group name for a number of related compounds, which have in common a methylated naphthoquinone ring structure, and which vary in the aliphatic side chain attached at the 3-position (see fig. 1). In this paper we will distinguish phylloquinone (also known as vitamin K_1), menaquinone-4 (MK-4) and the long-chain menaquinones (MK-n). It is generally accepted that the naphthoquinone is the functional group, so that the mechanism of action is similar for all K vitamins. Substantial differences may be expected, however, with respect to intestinal absorption, transport, tissue distribution, and bioavailability. These differences are caused by the different lipophilicity of the various side chains, and have been demonstrated by several authors in experimental animal studies [1–5]. Long-chain menaquinones, like MK-9, appear to be poorly absorbed [5], and at equimolar hepatic concentrations of phylloquinone and MK-4 the rate of utilization is 4:1 [2]. Because of the long biological half-life times, however, the effect of MK-9 extends over much longer periods than that of phylloquinone [3, 4].

Function of Vitamin K

In mammals the only known function of vitamin K is that it serves as a cofactor for γ-glutamylcarboxylase, an endoplasmic enzyme involved in the posttranslational carboxylation of glutamate residues into γ-carboxyglutamate (Gla). Hence, the vitamin K-dependent step is a carboxylation reaction (see fig. 2). The resulting Gla residues are found in a limited number of proteins, and in these proteins only at certain well-defined positions [6, 7]. Via specific staining [8] or HPLC detection techniques [9] these so-called Gla proteins can

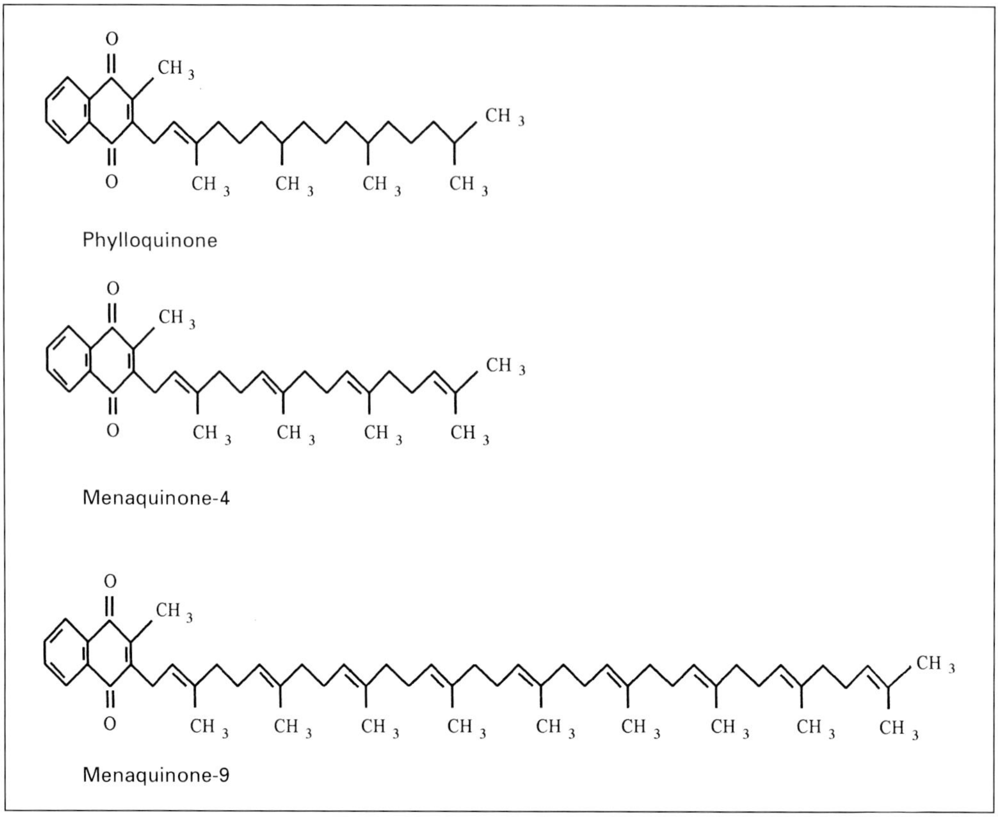

Fig. 1. Structures of different forms of vitamin K.

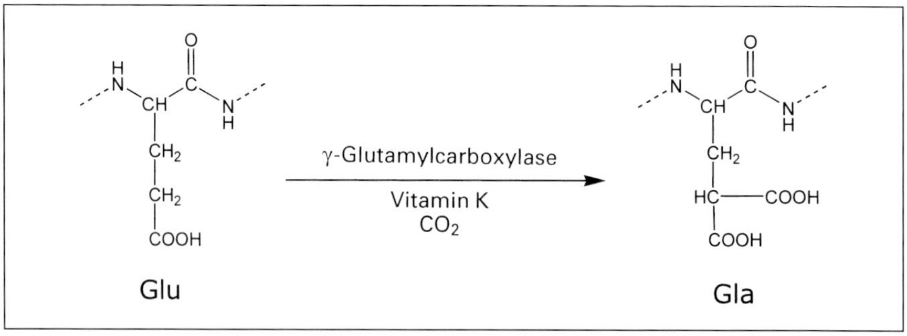

Fig. 2. The vitamin K-dependent carboxylation reaction.

Table 1. Vitamin K concentrations (ng/g) in foods on the Dutch market

Nutrient	K_1	MK-4	MK-9
Meat	5–30	10–80	0–10
Fish	1–0	1–16	0–15
Milk	5–10	2–20	0–20
Yoghurt	2–5	5–10	1–2
Cheese	25–150	50–100	400–800
Butter	90–200	100–200	0
Margarines (from plant oil)	800–1,100	0	0
Green vegetables	1,000–7,500	0	0
Fruit	1–30	0	0
Bread	5–10	0	0

Vitamin K was analyzed by HPLC using a C-18 reversed-phase column and fluorometric detection after post-column electrochemical reduction as was described previously [52]. Vitamin K_1 and menaquinones were determined in the same run. Authentic menaquinones (MK-4 through MK-10) were kindly supplied by F. Hoffmann-La Roche Ltd (Basel) and served as reference material. In all cases the range was determined after the analysis of 5–10 different samples.

be identified as unique products of vitamin K action. In case of vitamin K deficiency the carboxylation reaction cannot proceed, hence the Gla proteins are released in the circulation in an undercarboxylated form. These so-called descarboxy proteins were shown to be inactive in all cases in which the function of the corresponding Gla protein is known [10]. Gla residues form calcium-binding groups in proteins, so the main physicochemical difference between normal and descarboxy proteins is their large difference in both binding of calcium from solution and the adsorption of these proteins to insoluble calcium salts.

Sources of Vitamin K

By far the most abundant form of dietary vitamin K is phylloquinone (vitamin K_1), which occurs in green vegetables such as kale, spinach, broccoli and brussels sprouts [11]. Except for some plant oils [12], other foods have far lower phylloquinone contents (table 1). Other forms of vitamin K (menaquinones) are predominantly found in cheese, but in relatively low amounts, however. Also, the intestinal flora in the colon produces menaquinones, notably

MK-7, MK-8 and MK-9. These highly lipophilic compounds are tightly bound to the bacterial membranes, and require bile salts for their solubilization and absorption. Since virtually all cholate is absorbed in the small intestine, it is questionable whether the colonic pool of menaquinones contributes significantly to the human vitamin K status [13, 14]. This view is supported by experimental animal data showing that in rats, originally thought to be resistant to dietary deprivation, deficiency of vitamin K can be readily induced by preventing coprophagy [15]. Apparently rats can only utilize enterically synthesized menaquinones by a second passage through the bowel and presumably absorption from the upper region of the small bowel [14].

Human volunteer studies have shown that the absorption of phylloquinone from vegetables is low (between 3 and 10%), and depends on the concomitant fat intake [16]. The poor bioavailability of plant phylloquinone may be explained by its tight association with the chloroplasts. In contrast, the efficacy of absorption from pharmaceutical vitamin K_1 concentrates, such as the detergent-solubilized Konakion™ or Mixed Micelles™, is much higher (>80%) [16]. Although it has been demonstrated that after oral ingestion also the higher menaquinones can be utilized in humans, insufficient data are available about the efficacy of their absorption [17].

Functions of Gla Proteins

Vitamin K-dependent proteins are known to participate in three physiological processes: blood coagulation, bone metabolism and vascular biology. Gla proteins involved in these respective processes are: (a) *in blood:* the procoagulant proteins prothrombin, factors VII, IX and X, and the anticoagulant proteins C and S; (b) *in bone:* protein S, osteocalcin, and matrix Gla protein (MGP), and (c) *in arterial vessel wall:* protein S, MGP and growth arrest-specific protein 6 (Gas6).

Its involvement in blood coagulation is the classical role of vitamin K, and will not be discussed in this paper. Instead, we will focus on the Gla proteins synthesized in bone and vessel wall, and we will address the question whether the nutritonal vitamin K intake is sufficient to cover the requirements of these tissues.

Vitamin K and Bone Metabolism

All three bone Gla proteins are synthesized by the osteoblasts (the bone-forming cells), but only osteocalcin is a unique product of bone tissue. Protein

S and MGP are also synthesized in a number of soft tissues including the vessel wall (see below). Osteocalcin forms about 20% of the noncollagenous proteins in bone and is one of the most abundant proteins in humans. After its synthesis it is secreted by the osteoblasts and a major part is directly bound to the hydroxyapatite matrix of the bone. About 25% of the de novo synthesized osteocalcin, however, is set free in the circulation where it can be detected with commercially available test kits [18, 19]. So the serum concentration of osteocalcin forms a reflection of the osteoblast activity, which makes it an important and widely used marker for bone formation.

The importance of Gla proteins in bone became clear about 25 years ago. Since the end of the Second World War, vitamin K antagonists (coumarin derivatives) were used for the treatment of patients at risk for thromboembolic events. These drugs are powerful antagonists of vitamin K and are generally administered for periods of several years or longer. A major area of application was in the prevention of myocardial reinfarction. Most of these patients are well over 50 years of age. In the early 1970s, however, it became gradually more usual to treat also younger patients with coumarin derivatives, for instance in those having received an artificial heart valve. Because of compelling medical indications the treatment of women was continued even after they had become pregnant. It appeared, however, that in about 30% of the cases the newborns had developed serious bone defects [20]. Subsequent experiments in animals (rats, lambs) have shown that notably in rapidly growing (young) bone tissue, coumarin derivatives interfere with the regulation of calcium deposition resulting in excessive and irregular precipitation of calcium salts in areas which are normally not calcified (e.g. the growth plates). This leads to bone deformations and growth reduction [21–23]. Remarkably, coumarin derivatives appear to have less efects on adult bone [24–26].

The precise function of the three bone Gla proteins is not yet clear. Osteocalcin-deficient (so-called 'gene knockout') mice turned out to grow more rapidly than the wild types, but after ovariectomy their bones were more sensitive for estrogen deficiency, so that the reduction of bone mass was quicker than normal [27]. This may be of importance for postmenopausal women, whose estrogen production has also stopped almost completely leading to an increased bone resorption rate. If – like in rodents – osteocalcin would contribute to protecting against this form of bone loss in humans, it should be checked whether the daily vitamin K intake adequately covers the requirement of bone tissue. Knockout mice have also been generated for MGP. These animals showed substantial growth retardation, with excessive calcifications of their growth plates, osteopenia and bone fractures [28]. Since all animals died from cardiovascular disease within 2 months after birth (see below), long-term effects of MGP deficiency on bone are still unknown.

Vitamin K and Vascular Mineralization

In the arterial vessel wall the functions of Gla proteins are probably associated with: local inhibition of thrombosis (protein S), inhibition of mineralization (MGP), and stimulation of normal cell growth and prevention of apoptosis in growth-arrested cells (Gas6). As was discussed above, MGP-deficient mice were born to term but showed strongly impaired bone growth (–40%) and all died before the 8th week of life due to massive arterial calcification and rupture of the aorta. Excessive aorta mineralization was also observed in rats after 4–6 weeks of treatment with vitamin K antagonists [53]. Gla proteins have been extracted from human atheromatous plaques and although they were only characterized incompletely, the poor solubility of the human vascular Gla proteins indicates that the major fraction may be similar to MGP [29].

The function of Gas6 has only been investigated in cell culture systems thus far. In response to conditions leading to cell death, for instance during serum starvation, cells are induced to produce growth arrest-specific proteins. Most of these proteins promote cell death (apoptosis), but Gas6 is an exception in this respect: it was shown to prevent serum starvation-induced death of fibroblasts and smooth muscle cells, and also may act as a growth-potentiating factor which acts synergistically with other known growth factors in these cells [30, 31]. Gla residues were shown to be essential for its functions in cell culture. Data presently available suggest that in humans Gas6 may play a key role in preventing the degeneration of an atherosclerotic vessel wall.

Assessment of Human Vitamin K Status

As has been explained above, the occurrence of descarboxy proteins in the circulation has enabled us to develop biochemical tests to monitor human vitamin K status, and to screen for vitamin K deficiency. In this respect, vitamin K is unique among the vitamins. Already in 1991 it was found in population-based studies that circulating osteocalcin is far more sensitive for poor vitamin K status than other Gla proteins are [32]. There are two mechanisms underlying this observation. First, the affinity for γ-glutamylcarboxylase of the endoplasmic osteocalcin precursor proteins (pro-osteocalcin) is distinctly lower than that of other Gla proteins. It was demonstrated that this poor affinity is due to an Ala^{-10}→Gly mutation in the leader sequence: during periods of poor vitamin K supply precursor proteins will accumulate, and the competition for the carboxylase-binding site will inevitably be lost by pro-osteocalcin [33]. Second, after its synthesis by the osteoblasts, osteocalcin is set free amidst the hydroxyapatite matrix of bone, which will preferentially adsorb the normally carboxylated osteocalcin, so that undercarboxylated osteocalcin will be selectively set free in the circulation. We propose to define mild vitamin K deficiency as a condition in which the circulating osteocalcin is significantly undercarboxylated, whereas the blood coagulation factor prothrombin is normal. Severe vitamin K deficiency may then be regarded as a condition in which descarboxyprothrombin is detectable in the circulation.

Groups at Risk for Vitamin K Deficiency

Severe vitamin K deficiency with elevated levels of descarboxyprothrombin may be found in newborns [14, 34, 35]. Therefore, babies are at risk of developing the hemorrhagic disease of the newborn (HDN), and require vitamin K prophylaxis at birth [36]. Moreover, human milk contains insufficient vitamin K to meet recommended intakes for infants below 6 months of age [37, 38]. In most countries, guidelines have been published to supplement newborns with vitamin K either as a food supplement (in case of breastfeeding) or as fortified food (formula milk).

Whereas undercarboxylated prothrombin is rarely detectable in healthy adults, undercarboxylated osteocalcin is rather common, notably in the elderly [39–41]. The undercarboxyated osteocalcin was shown to be responsive to vitamin K supplementation: circulating levels rapidly decreased upon vitamin K administration [39, 40]. According to the above definition, these subjects must be regarded as being mildly vitamin K-deficient. Because the circulating levels of the vitamin K-dependent coagulation factors were not affected, it appears that hemostasis may be normal, whereas other physiological functions, like osteblast activity and bone metabolism, are impaired. Below we will summarize the available literature data suggesting a correlation between vitamin K status and bone metabolism.

In 1984 it was shown by the group of Shearer [42] that 16 subsequent osteoporotic patients with femur neck fractures had circulating vitamin K_1 levels which were less than 30% of those in 34 controls. In a subsequent study from the same group it was confirmed that in osteoporotic hip fractures and in spinal crush fractures the circulating vitamin K concentrations were 21 and 24% of the matched controls, respectively [43]. Similar data were observed by the group of Delmas [44], who showed that besides vitamin K_1 also circulating menaquinones were strongly reduced in elderly women with hip fractures. It remained to be proven, however, that the low circulating vitamin K concentrations were indicative for poor vitamin K status in the bone tissue. In 1989 it was reported by Knapen et al. [39] that high levels of undercarboxylated osteocalcin were detectable in serum from postmenopausal women, and that they were reduced upon supplementation with a vitamin K concentrate. The data, which strongly suggest that a mild vitamin K deficiency is common in elderly women, were confirmed by the group of Delmas [41] who also showed that circulating undercarboxylated osteocalcin is inversely correlated with bone mass [45], and that it is a strong risk factor for hip fracture [46, 47]. Further evidence for the vitamin K deficiency of human bone came from the group of Price [48], who isolated osteocalcin from the femoral heads removed during hip replacement surgery in elderly subjects suffering from osteoporotic fractures or degenerative joint disease. The authors concluded that their studies provide strong support to the view that there is a widespread undercarboxylation of osteocalcin in humans, a defect that may reflect inadequate levels of vitamin K in bone cells.

Vitamin K Supplementation Studies

In light of the conclusions above it seemed indicated to investigate whether increased intake of vitamin K might positively influence bone metabolism. Thus far, all studies have focused on effects of vitamin K supplementation in postmenopausal women. Because of economical reasons, studies on the effects of new drugs on fracture risk are generally preceded by trials in which the effects on bone markers and on bone mass are monitored. A substantial amount of information is presently available on effects of vitamin K on bone markers, limited data have been reported on its effects on bone mass (although at least two clinical trials are in progress), whereas effects on fracture risk have not been evaluated at this time. It has been confirmed in several placebo-controlled trials that the daily intake of 1–10 mg/day of vitamin K_1 (in the form of a pharmaceutical concentrate) results in an increase of serum markers for bone formation (bone-specific alkaline phosphatase, osteocalcin total antigen), and in an increase of urine markers for bone resorption (hydroxyproline, deoxypyridinoline) [39–41]. Also urinary calcium loss was decreased, notably in those with high calcium excretion [39, 40, 50]. These data suggest that increased vitamin K intake may favorably affect the balance between bone formation and bone resorption in elderly women.

Studies concerning the effect of vitamin K supplements on bone mass have only been completed in Japan. Although the authors claim that in all cases postmenopausal bone loss is substantially reduced [49, 50], and in some cases bone mass is even increased [50], we should keep in mind that Japanese women differ from Caucasians in many aspects including their genetic disposition, food intake and lifestyle. The average calcium intake among Japanese women, for instance, is as low as 300 mg/day. The effects observed among Japanese women need therefore not be valid in other populations. Several intervention studies measuring bone mass have started in Europe and the USA this year, but data may not be expected within 2 years from now. No data are available on the possible effects of increased vitamin K intake on vascular biology.

Potential Side Effects of High Vitamin K Intake

Since for many decades vitamin K has been exclusively associated with blood coagulation, and because vitamin K deficiency leads to bleeding, it is often argued that high vitamin K intake might give rise to an increased thrombosis tendency. This is not the case, however. First, the rate at which Gla proteins are synthesized in the liver is not under the influence of vitamin K. Second, the number of carboxylatable glutamate residues in coagulation factor precursors is limited (10–12 per molecule), and both in vivo and in vitro carboxylation remains restricted to these well-defined sites. Neither in experimental animals nor in humans have high vitamin K intakes (up to 5,000 × RDA) led to increased levels of coagulation factors, increased procoagulant activity or blood platelet activity [51].

Human Vitamin K Requirement

As was mentioned above, newborns are at risk of developing vitamin K deficiency, and supplementation is recommended in most countries. Although various national health policies may vary to some extent, the most appropriate dose seems to be 25 μg/day. RDA values for vitamin K in adults are only given in the USA and the UK, and are based on the requirement for optimal hepatic clotting factor synthesis (1 μg/day · kg body weight). For healthy adults this amounts to 60–80 μg/day, which is equivalent to the contents of about 15 g of spinach. From the discussion above it appears that the requirement for extrahepatic functions of vitamin K may be substantially higher. Based on the data presently available it is justified to conclude that the nutritional vitamin K intake, notably in elderly, is marginal and that a mean intake of 500 μg/day (equivalent to about 100 g of green vegetables) is desirable. In case this amount is not met, food supplements containing 50 μg/day would be sufficient to increase a subject's vitamin K status to a comparable level. It is unlikely that the proposed dosages will interfere with oral anticoagulant therapy, but this point needs to be addressed before a formal recommendation can be given.

Conclusions

Vitamin K-dependent proteins play a regulatory role in at least three important physiological processes: blood coagulation, bone metabolism and vascular biology. All data presently available suggest that for normal hemostasis the nutritional vitamin K intake is adequate, but that both other functions may require intakes above the RDA levels presently accepted in some countries. Long-term low vitamin K intake may be associated with postmenopausal osteoporosis and with vascular mineralization (atherosclerosis). No RDA levels have been defined in any European country except Great Britain, but public health care requires that quick decisions will be taken in this respect, preferrably on a supernational level.

References

1 Will BH, Suttie JW: Comparative metabolism of phylloquinone and menaquinone-9 in rat liver. J Nutr 1992;122:953–958.
2 Reedstrom CK, Suttie JW: Comparative distribution, metabolism, and utilization of phylloquinone and menaquinone-9 in the rat liver. Proc Soc Exp Biol Med 1995;209:403–409.
3 Groenen-van Dooren MMCL, Soute BAM, Jie KSG, Thijssen HHW, Vermeer C: The relative effects of phylloquinone and menaquinone on the blood coagulation factor synthesis in vitamin K-deficient rats. Biochem Pharmacol 1993;46:433–437.
4 Groenen-van Dooren MMCL, Ronden JE, Soute BAM, Vermeer C: Bioavailability of phylloquinone and menaquinones after oral and colorectal administration in the vitamin K-deficient rat. Biochem Pharmacol 1995;50:797–801.
5 Crăciun AM, Groenen-van Dooren MMCL, Thijssen HHW, Vermeer C: Induction of prothrombin synthesis by K-vitamins compared in vitamin K-deficient and in brodifacoum-treated rats. Biochim Biophys Acta 1998;1380:75–81.
6 Furie B, Furie BC: Molecular basis of vitamin K-dependent γ-carboxylation. Blood 1990;75:1753–1762.
7 Vermeer C: Gamma-carboxyglutamate-containing proteins and the vitamin K-dependent carboxylase. Biochem J 1990;266:625–636.
8 Jie KSG, Gijsbers BLMG, Vermeer C: A specific colorimetric staining method for γ-carboxyglutamic acid-containing proteins in polyacrylamide gels. Analyt Biochem 1995;224:163–165.
9 Kuwada M, Katayama K: An improved method for determination of γ-carboxyglutamic acid in proteins, bone and urine. Analyt Biochem 1983;131:173–179.
10 Vermeer C, Hamulyák K: Pathophysiology of vitamin K deficiency and oral anticoagulants. Thromb Haemost 1991;66:153–159.
11 Booth SL, Sadowski JA, Weihrauch JL, Ferland G: Vitamin K_1 (phylloquinone) content of foods: A provisional table. J Food Comp Anal 1993;6:109–120.
12 Ferland G, Sadowski JA: Vitamin K_1 (phylloquinone) content of edible oils: Effects of heating and light exposure. J Agric Food Chem 1992;40:1869–1873.
13 Conly JM, Stein K, Worobetz L, Rutledge-Harding S: The contribution of vitamin K2 (menaquinones) produced by intestinal microflora to human nutritional requirements for vitamin K. Am J Gastroenterol 1994;89:915–923.
14 Shearer MJ: Vitamin K metabolism and nutriture. Blood Rev 1992;6:92–104.
15 Barnes RH, Fiala G: Effects of the prevention of coprophagy in the rat. VI. Vitamin K. J Nutr 1959;68:603–614.

16 Shearer MJ, McBurney A, Barkhan P: Studies on the absorption and metabolism of phylloquinone (vitamin K_1) in man. Vitam Horm 1974;32:513–542.
17 Conly JM, Stein K: The absorption and bioactivity of bacterially synthesized menaquinones. Clin Invest Med 1993;16:45–57.
18 Power MJ, Fottrell PF: Osteocalcin: Diagnostic methods and clinical applications. Crit Rev Clin Lab Sci 1991;28:287–335.
19 Knapen MHJ, Eisenwiener HG, Vermeer C: Osteocalcin detection in aging serum and whole blood: Stability of different osteocalcin fractions. Clin Chim Acta 1996;256:151–164.
20 Pettifor JM, Benson R: Congenital malformations associated with the administration of oral anticoagulants during pregnancy. J Pediatr 1975;86:459–462.
21 Price PA, Williamson MK, Haba T, Dell RB, Jee WS: Excessive mineralization with growth plate closure in rats on chronic warfarin treatment. Proc Natl Acad Sci USA 1982;79:7734–7738.
22 Howe AM, Webster WS: The warfarin embryopathy: A rat model showing maxillonasal hypoplasia and other skeletal disturbances. Teratology 1992;46:379–390.
23 Pastoureau P, Vergnaud P, Meunier PJ, Delmas PD: Ostopenia and bone-remodeling abnormalities in warfarin-treated lambs. J Bone Miner Res 1993;8:1417–1426.
24 Rosen HN, Maitland LA, Suttie JW, Manning WJ, Glynn RJ, Greenspan SL: Vitamin K and maintenance of skeletal integrity in adults. Am J Med 1993;94:62–68.
25 Fiore CE, Tamburino C, Foti R, Grimaldi D: Reduced bone mineral content in patients taking an oral anticoagulant. South Med J 1990;83:538–542.
26 Resch H, Pietschmann P, Krexner E, Willvonseder R: Decreased peripheral bone mineral content in patients under anticoagulant therapy with phenprocoumon. Eur Heart J 1991;12:439–441.
27 Ducy P, Desbois C, Boyce B, Pinero G, Story B, Dunstan C, Smith E, Bonadio J, Goldstein S, Gundberg C, Bradley A, Karsenty G: Increased bone formation in osteocalcin-deficient mice. Nature 1996;382:448–452.
28 Luo G, Ducy P, McKee MD, Pinero GJ, Loyer E, Behringer RR, Karsenty G: Spontaneous calcification of arteries and cartilage in mice lacking matrix GLA protein. Nature 1997;386:78–81.
29 Gijsbers BLMG, van Haarlem LJM, Soute BAM, Ebberink RHM, Vermeer C: Characterization of a Gla-containing protein from calcified human atherosclerotic plaques. Arteriosclerosis 1990;10: 991–995.
30 Nakano T, Kawamoto K, Kishino J, Nomura K, Higashino K, Arita H: Requirement of γ-carboxyglutamic acid residues for the biological activity of Gas6: Contribution of endogenous Gas6 to the proliferation of vascular smooth muscle cells. Biochem J 1997;323:387–392.
31 Goruppi S, Ruaro E, Schneider C: Gas6, the ligand of Axl tyrosine kinase receptor, has mitogenic and survival activities for serum starved NIH3T3 fibroblasts. Oncogene 1996;12:471–480.
32 Knapen MHJ, Jie KSG, Hamulyák K, Vermeer C: Vitamin K deficiency redefined. Thromb Haemost 1991;65:671.
33 Chu K, Wu SM, Stanley T, Stafford DW, High KA: A mutation in the propeptide of factor IX leads to warfarin sensitivity by a novel mechanism. J Clin Invest 1996;98:1619–1625.
34 Greer F: Vitamin K deficiency and hemorrhage in infancy. Clin Perinat 1995;22:759–777.
35 Von Kries R, Greer FR, Suttie JW: Assessment of vitamin K status of the newborn infant. J Pediatr Gastroenterol Nutr 1993;16:231–238.
36 Von Kries R: Vitamin K prophylaxis – A useful public health measure? Paediatr Perinat Epidemiol 1992;6:7–13.
37 Canfield LM, Hopkinson JM, Lima AF, Silva AF, Garza C: Vitamin K in colostrum and mature human milk over the lactation period – A cross-sectional study. Am J Clin Nutr 1991;53:730–735.
38 Greer FR, Marshall S, Cherry J, Suttie JW: Vitamin K status of lactating mothers, human milk, and breast-feeding infants. Pediatrics 1991;88:751–756.
39 Knapen MHJ, Hamulyák K, Vermeer C: The effect of vitamin K supplementation on circulating osteocalcin (bone Gla protein) and urinary calcium excretion. Ann Intern Med 1989;111:1001–1005.
40 Knapen MHJ, Jie KSG, Hamulyák K, Vermeer C: Vitamin K-induced changes in markers for osteoblast activitiy and urinary calcium loss. Calcif Tissue Int 1993;53:81–85.
41 Plantalech L, Guillaumont M, Vergnaud P, Leclercq M, Delmas PD: Impairment of γ-carboxylation of circulating osteocalcin (bone Gla protein) in elderly women. J Bone Miner Res 1991;6:1211–1216.

42 Hart JP, Catterall A, Dodds RA, Klenerman L, Shearer MJ, Bitensky L, Chayen J: Circulating vitamin K_1 levels in fractured neck of femur. Lancet 1984;ii:283.
43 Hart JP, Shearer MJ, Klenerman L, Caterall A, Reeve J, Sambrook PN, Dodds RA, Bitensky L, Chayen J: Electrochemical detection of depressed circulating levels of vitamin K_1 in osteoporosis. J Clin Endocrinol Metab 1985;60:1268–1269.
44 Hodges SJ, Akesson K, Vergnaud P, Obrant K, Delmas PD: Circulating levels of vitamins K_1 and K_2 decreased in elderly women with hip fracture. J Bone Miner Res 1993;8:1241–1245.
45 Szulc P, Arlot M, Chapuy MC, Duboeuf F, Meunier PJ, Delmas PD: Serum undercarboxylated osteocalcin correlates with hip bone mineral density in elderly women. J Bone Miner Res 1994;9:1591–1595.
46 Szulc P, Chapuy MC, Meunier PJ, Delmas PD: Serum undercarboxylated osteocalcin is a marker of the risk of hip fracture in elderly women. J Clin Invest 1993;91:1769–1774.
47 Szulc P, Chapuy MC, Meunier PJ, Delmas PD: Serum undercarboxylated osteocalcin is a marker of the risk of hip fracture: A three-year follow-up study. Bone 1996;18:487–488.
48 Cairns JR, Price PA: Direct demonstration that the vitamin K-dependent bone Gla protein is incompletely γ-carboxylated in humans. J Bone Miner Res 1994;9:1989–1997.
49 Akiba T, Kurihara S, Tachibana K, Kuwahara M, Sakamoto H, Yoneshima H, Marumo F: Vitamin K increased bone mass in hemodialysis patients with low-turnover bone disease. J Am Soc Nephrol 1991;2:608.
50 Orimo H, Shiraki M, Fujita T, Onomura T, Inoue T, Kushida K: Clinical evaluation of menatetrenone in the treatment of involutional osteoporosis – A double-blind multicenter comparative study with 1α-hydroxyvitamin D_3. J Bone Miner Res 1992;7:S122.
51 Ronden JE, Groenen-van Dooren MMCL, Hornstra G, Vermeer C: Modulation of arterial thrombosis tendency in rats by vitamin K and its side chains. Atherosclerosis 1997;132:61–67.
52 Gijsbers BLMG, Jie KSG, Vermeer C: Effect of food composition on vitamin K absorption in human volunteers. Br J Nutr 1996;76:223–229.
53 Price PA, Faus SA, Williamson MK: Warfarin causes rapid calcification of the elastic lamellae in rat arteries and heart valves. Arterioscler Thromb Vasc Biol 1998;18:1400–1407.

Dr. C. Vermeer, Department of Biochemistry, Cardiovascular Research Institute,
University of Limburg, NL-6200 MD Maastricht (The Netherlands)
Tel. +31 43 388 1682, Fax +31 43 367 0992, E-Mail c.vermeer@bioch.unimaas.nl

Walter P, Hornig D, Moser U (eds): Functions of Vitamins beyond Recommended Dietary Allowances. Bibl Nutr Dieta. Basel, Karger, 2001, No 55, pp 171–176

Behavioural and Mental Functions

Hannes B. Stähelin

Geriatric University Clinic, Kantonsspital, Basel, Switzerland

Mental symptoms such as cognitive impairment, emotional irritability or neurological signs are well known in vitamin deficiencies. If unrecognized, these conditions may lead to irreversible disabilities [1]. There is evidence that above average intake of vitamins and other micronutrients could delay or even prevent the occurrence of degenerative disorders. Chronic diseases are an increasing burden in an increasingly ageing society. Thus, the prospect of postponing or even preventing the onset of disability due to cognitive impairment is of central importance in today's health policy. Mental impairment as a result of chronic degenerative brain disease has a particularly severe impact on autonomy. Thus, effective preventive strategies against illnesses causing dementia and related neurological disorders are urgently needed.

This chapter explores epidemiological data relating vitamin intake to mental and behavioural functions and looks into suggested pathophysiological hypotheses that could explain the observed association between micronutrients and health outcome.

Conceptually, we will distinguish between probable direct effects on cells of the central nervous system and effects influencing circulation and hence the nutrient and oxygen supply of the brain tissue.

Vascular Disease

Large geographical variations clearly relate atherosclerosis of coronary and brain vessels to environmental factors. The impressive decline in stroke and cardiovascular disease [2] over the last three decades is in part related to active treatment of risk factors, but probably even more so to improved nutrition, particularly the intake of antioxidant micronutrients. The striking 4-fold

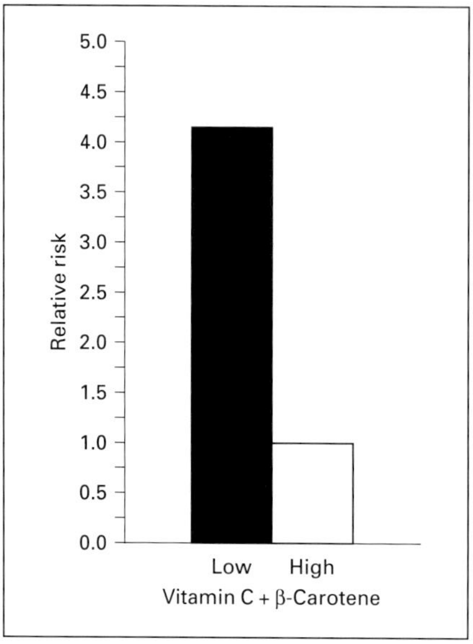

Fig. 1. In the Basel Study, combined low plasma levels of β-carotene and vitamin C were associated with significant increased risk for stroke.

higher stroke mortality (fig. 1) in subjects with simultaneously low plasma concentration of vitamin C and carotene ($<$quartile 1) demonstrates that concentrations already at plasma levels in the low normal range increase the risk for vascular diseases [3]. It is now well recognized that a high cardiovascular risk correlates with a high stroke risk and thus with vascular dementia. In the study by Gale et al. [4], stroke was associated with low vitamin C intake, and cognitive impairment was associated with stroke. This demonstrates very nicely the close relationship between stroke and vascular dementia, which share also common risk factors such as hypertension, smoking, diabetes mellitus, atrial fibrillation and, to a lesser extent, hyperlipidaemia [5–7]. Homocysteine levels might be important, linking folic acid, vitamins B_6 and B_{12} with vascular dementia [8, 9].

Cognitive Impairment in Elderly Subjects

A number of earlier studies reported better performance in cognitive tests in subjects with higher plasma levels or intake of a variety of vitamins. Thus, both Goodwin et al. [10] and Chome et al. [11] found an association between micronutrient intake and cognitive performance. More recent studies analyzed different nutrients with regard to cognition in elderly subjects. In one such study, Wahlin et al. [12] observed better cognitive function in subjects with

Table 1. The relation between antioxidants and memory performance in the old and very old: intercorrelations of antioxidants, blood pressure, plasma cholesterol and plasma ferritin adjusted for age, sex and smoking

	Priming[1]	WM[2]	Free-recall	Recognition	Wais-R[3]
Vitamin C, 1971	–0.02	0.02	0.01	0.04	0.11*
Vitamin C, 1993	–0.05	0.03	0.10*	0.06	0.16**
β-Carotene, 1971	0.05	0.06	0.05	0.12*	0.10*
β-Carotene, 1993	–0.04	0.00	0.13**	0.22**	0.14**
Vitamin E, 1971	0.06	0.00	–0.02	0.02	0.09
Vitamin E, 1993	0.07	0.05	0.05	0.08	0.04
Blood pressure, 1993	0.04	–0.01	–0.03	0.07	–0.01
Plasma cholesterol, 1993	–0.01	–0.03	0.04	0.13**	–0.02
Plasma ferritin, 1993	0.02	0.00	–0.13**	–0.14**	–0.01

[1] Priming: implicit memory. [2] WM: working memory. [3] Wais-R: semantic memory.
*$p<0.05$. **$p<0.01$.

vitamin B_{12} levels >200 pmol/l compared to lower levels. They concluded that subjects with intakes or plasma levels at the lower end perform less well compared to subjects with normal levels. They concluded that normal levels are sufficient for normal cognitive function, and subnormal levels may be associated with cognitive impairment.

Brain ageing is associated with oxidative stress; thus, antioxidants are of particular interest. The prospective Basel Study with a complete plasma vitamin analysis in 1971–1973 [13] allows a long-term follow-up, since in 1993, 452 participants aged 65 or older took part in a study focusing on cognitive changes during ageing [14]. The observed correlation between biological parameters and memory function is given in table 1. It is noteworthy that neither smoking nor blood pressure was predictive, but high plasma vitamin C and β-carotene, even if measured 20 years before the tests, predicted better memory performance. One concern in this kind of study is the fact that better education and socioeconomic status might lead to better memory performance and simultaneously better micronutrient intake. As figure 2 shows, the relationship is maintained even if we look at the different educational levels, comparing low plasma levels (below median) versus high (above median). We therefore concluded that educational levels, albeit of great importance, are not strong enough to explain the observed differences.

The findings of the Basel Study population, where β-carotene plasma concentrations correlate with memory performance, is in agreement with

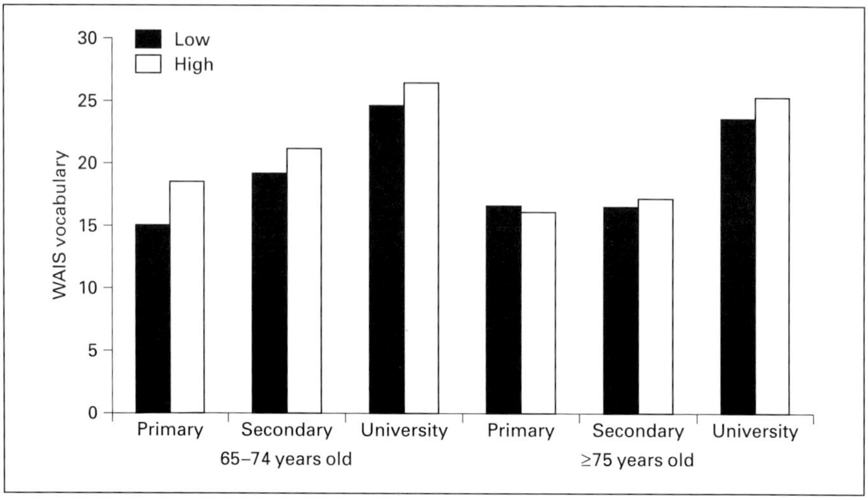

Fig. 2. Plasma vitamin C, age, education, and semantic memory. WAIS vocabulary = Wechsler Adult Intelligence Scale: Vocabulary subtest.

Table 2. Correlation between plasma micronutrients and cognition (MMSE) SENECA data [16]

Total carotene	0.097**
α-Carotene	0.11***
β-Carotene	0.089**
Lycopene	0.174***
β-Cryptoxanthin	0.194***
Cobalamin	0.125***
Folate	0.103*
α-Tocopherol	0.156***

*p < 0.05, **p < 0.01, ***p < 0.001.

results from the Rotterdam Study [15]. There, low intake of β-carotene (≤0.9 mg/day) was associated with significantly poorer cognitive performance when compared to subjects with an intake of ≥2.1 mg/day. In the SENECA-EURONUT Investigation [16], subjects from European towns born between 1911 and 1914 were analyzed. It was remarkable that the plasma carotene, vitamin C and α-tocopherol concentrations correlated with the MMSE, a screening method of cognitive function to detect dementing disorders (table 2). Of great interest is the observation of de Rijk et al. [17] who suggests that a high intake of dietary vitamin E may protect against the occurrence of Parkinson's disease.

Taken together, these data strongly suggest that carotene and carotenoids, ascorbic acid and α-tocopherol influence brain ageing. In contrast to cardiovascular disease, no clear evidence is available to suggest additional benefits by intakes above RDAs. Primary preventive intervention trials showing a benefit in delaying cognitive decline over time are not yet available. On theoretical grounds, a slowing down of deterioration might be expected, which is rather difficult to demonstrate in the absence of overt degenerative brain disease.

Micronutrients in Secondary Prevention and Treatment of Degenerative Brain Disease

A review of the literature reveals only a very limited number of studies. Systematic studies investigating the effect of high doses of vitamin in primary degenerative dementias are rare. The preliminary finding of a favourable effect of very high thiamin dosages (3–8 g/day) in Alzheimer's disease were not followed further [18]. The identification of free radical involvement in Parkinson's disease formed the rationale of the study by Fahn et al. [19, 20]. This research group evaluated the effect of high doses of vitamin E and ascorbic acid. In 1992, they reported that intake of 1,800 IU of vitamin E and ascorbate delayed the necessity of dopa substitution by 2.4 years. This work remains, however, unconfirmed. In addition, it is not clarified whether vitamin E in such high amounts acts only as antioxidant or whether effects on microcirculation or even pro-oxidant effects could be important. The probable protective effect of smoking on Parkinson's disease should not be overlooked.

A recent study in patients with mild to moderate Alzheimer's disease [21] again treating with 1,800 IU α-tocopherol found a significant slowing in the deterioration of mental function, leading to a delay in institutionalization compared to untreated controls. The therapeutic effect was comparable to the effect of selegilin therapy alone. Interestingly, the combination of selegilin and α-tocopherol did not increase treatment efficacy. Again, the same caveats apply as in Parkinson's disease for this study. Furthermore, the high dose of vitamin E was not accompanied by an additional increased intake of ascorbic acid.

Nevertheless, the pathophysiological rationale of antioxidants and B vitamins in chronic degenerative brain disease have opened new preventive and therapeutic possibilities to reduce and delay age-associated mental decline. It may well be that vitamins will contribute substantially to the maintenance of autonomy in old age.

References

1 Biesalski HK, Schrezenmeir J, Weber P, Weiss H: Vitamine. Physiologie, Pathophysiologie, Therapie. Stuttgart, Thieme, 1997.

2 Braunwald E: Shattuck lecture: Cardiovascular medicine at the turn of the millennium: Triumphs, concerns, and opportunities. N Engl J Med 1997;337:1360–1369.

3 Stähelin HB: Antioxidants and atherosclerosis; in Guesry P, Hennerici H, Sitzer G (eds): Nutrition and Stroke. Philadelphia, Lippincott-Raven, 1997.

4 Gale CR, Martyn CN, Cooper C: Cognitive impairment and mortality in a cohort of elderly people. BMJ 1996;312:608–611.

5 Skoog I: Risk factors for vascular dementia: A review. Dementia 1994;5:137–144.

6 Lai SM, Alter M, Friday G, Sobel E: A multifactorial analysis of risk factors for recurrence of ischemic stroke. Stroke 1994;25:958–962.

7 Yoshitake T, Kiyohara Y, Kato I, Ohmura T, Iwamoto H, Nakayama K, Ohmori S, Nomiyama K, Kawano H, Ueda K, Sueishi K, Tsuneyashi M, Fujishima M: Incidence and risk factors of vascular dementia and Alzheimer's disease in a defined elderly Japanese population: The Hisayama Study. Neurology 1995;45:1161–1168.

8 Koehler KM, Romero LJ, Stauber PM, Pareo TS, Liang HC, Baumgartner RN, Garry PJ, Allen RH, Stabler SP: Vitamin supplementation and other variables affecting serum homocysteine and methylmalonic acid concentrations in elderly men and women. J Am Coll Nutr 1996;15:364–376.

9 Bottiglieri T: Folate, vitamin B_{12}, and neuropsychiatric disorders. Nutr Rev 1996;54:382–390.

10 Goodwin JS, Goodwin JM, Garry PJ: Association between nutritional status and cognitive functioning in a healthy elderly population. JAMA 1982;249:2917–2921.

11 Chome J, Paul T, Pudel V, Bleyl H, Heseker H, Huppe R, Kubler W: Effects of suboptimal vitamin status on behavior. Bibl Nutr Dieta. Basel, Karger, 1986, pp 94–103.

12 Wahlin A, Hill RD, Winblad B, Backman L: Effects of serum vitamin B_{12} and folate status on episodic memory performance in very old age: A population-based study. Psychol Aging 1996;11:487–496.

13 Wildmer LK, Stähelin HB, Nissen C, da Silva A: Venen-, Arterienkrankheiten, koronare Herzkrankheit bei Berufstätigen ('Basler Studie'). Bern, Huber, 1981.

14 Perrig WJ, Perrig P, Stähelin HB: The relation between antioxidants and memory performance in the old and very old. J Am Geriatr Soc 1997;45:718–724.

15 Jama JW, Launer LJ, Witteman JC, den BJ, Breteler MM, Grobbee DE, Hofman A: Dietary antioxidants and cognitive function in a population-based sample of older persons. The Rotterdam Study. Am J Epidemiol 1996;144:275–280.

16 Haller J, Weggemans RM, Ferry M, Guigoz Y: Mental health: Mini-Mental State Examination and Geriatric Depression Score of elderly Europeans in the SENECA Study of 1993. Eur J Clin Nutr 1996;50(suppl 2):112–116.

17 de Rijk M, Breteler MM, den Breeijen J, Launer LJ, Grobbee DE, van der Meche F, Hofman A: Dietary antioxidants and Parkinson disease. The Rotterdam Study. Arch Neurol 1997;54:762–765.

18 Meador K, Loring D, Nichols M, Zamrini E, Rivner M, Posas H, Thompson E, Moore E: Preliminary findings of high-dose thiamine in dementia of Alzheimer's type. J Geriatr Psychiatry Neurol 1993;6:222–229.

19 Fahn S: A pilot trial of high-dose alpha-tocopherol and ascorbate in early Parkinson's disease. Ann Neurol 1992;32:S128–S132.

20 Fahn S, Cohen G: The oxidant stress hypothesis in Parkinson's disease: Evidence supporting it. Ann Neurol 1992;32:804–812.

21 Sano M, Ernesto C, Thomas RG, Klauber MR, Schafer K, Grundman M, Woodbury P, Growdon J, Cotman CW, Pfeiffer E, Schneider LS, Thal LJ: A controlled trial of selegiline, alpha-tocopherol, or both as treatment for Alzheimer's disease. the Alzheimer's Disease Cooperative Study. N Engl J Med 1997;336:1216–1222.

Hannes B. Stähelin, Geriatric University Clinic, Kantonsspital Basel,
CH–4031 Basel (Switzerland)
Tel. +41 61 265 2954, Fax +41 61 265 2670, E-Mail Hannes-B.Staehelin@unibas.ch

Walter P, Hornig D, Moser U (eds): Functions of Vitamins beyond Recommended Dietary Allowances. Bibl Nutr Dieta. Basel, Karger, 2001, No 55, pp 177–188

Vitamins and Regulation of Gene Expression

Angelo Azzi [a], *Elisabetta Aratri* [a], *Daniel Boscoboinik* [a], *Sophie Clément* [a], *Nesrin Özer* [b], *Roberta Ricciarelli* [a], *Stefan Spycher* [a], *Achim Stocker* [a]

[a] Institut für Biochemie und Molekularbiologie, Universität Bern, Schweiz and
[b] Department of Biochemistry, Marmara Medical School, Istanbul, Turkey

A number of vitamins have been reported to affect the regulation of gene expression. The most recent results on this subject will be critically reviewed with special focus on the effective dose in vivo, that may be extrapolated from in vitro studies.

Carotenoids, Vitamin A and Retinoids

all-trans-Retinoic acid (RA) is the major biologically active form of vitamin A, and nuclear retinoid receptors are the major mediators of *all-trans*-RA actions [1, 2]. RA metabolites of vitamin A are key regulators of gene expression involved in embryonic development and maintenance of epithelial tissues [3]. The absence of retinoic acid receptor (RAR) γ is associated with loss of the RA-inducible expression of the Hoxa-1, Hoxa-3, laminin B1, collagen IV (α_1), GATA-4, and BMP-2 genes. [4] Furthermore, the loss of RAR-γ is associated with a reduction in the metabolism of *all-trans*-RA to more polar derivatives, while the loss of RAR-α is associated with an increase in metabolism of RA [4]. RA also induces osteopontin gene expression in concert with vitamin D [5] and *all-trans*-RA 4-hydrolase [6] and suppresses that of collagenase [7]. Carotenoids both with and without provitamin A upregulate gap junctional communication and connexin43 gene expression in human dermal fibroblasts and inhibit carcinogen-induced neoplastic transformation [8, 9].

Vitamin C

The expression of alkaline phosphatase, type I collagen and osteocalcin are increased by ascorbic acid and are diminished in scurvy [10]. Calcineurin (protein phosphatase 2B) is an Fe^{2+} enzyme, that is inhibited by superoxide radicals and activated by ascorbate [11]. Since inactivation of calcineurin (by cyclosporin A or FK506) results in the inhibition of interleukin-2 gene expression, its specific (not obtained by other reducing agents) activation by ascorbate may be at the basis of an immune response enhancement by vitamin C [12].

Vitamin D

1,25 Dihydroxyvitamin D_3 interaction with the vitamin D receptor results not only in calcium homeostasis regulation, but has numerous other functions including inhibition of proliferation of cancer cells, effects on hormone secretion and suppression of T-cell proliferation and cytokine production. These effects are possibly related to gene expression regulation [13].

Vitamins K

The vitamins K were found to increase the expression of prothrombin and carboxylase messenger RNA and c-myc messenger RNA, but had no effect on the expression to TGF-β_1 messenger RNA [14, 15].

Vitamin E

Effect of α- and β-Tocopherol on Smooth Muscle Cell Proliferation

α-Tocopherol at concentrations between 10 and 50 μM (comparable to the physiological range of 25–40 μM), inhibits rat A7r5 smooth muscle cell proliferation (fig. 1A), while β-tocopherol is ineffective. When α- and β-tocopherol are added together, no inhibition of cell growth is seen. Both compounds are transported equally in cells and do not compete with each other for the uptake [16]. The oxidized product of α-tocopherol, α-tocopheryl quinone, and several other water-and lipid-soluble antioxidants are not inhibitory, indicating that the effects of α-tocopherol are not related to its antioxidant properties [16]. Inhibitory effects of α-tocopherol are also observed in primary human aortic smooth muscle cells (hAOMSC from Clonetics Corp.,

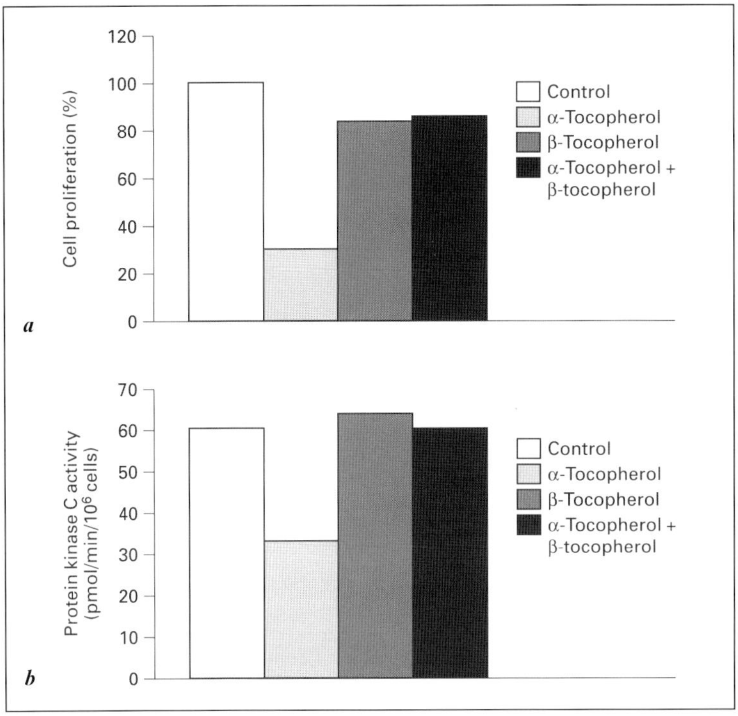

Fig. 1. Differential effects of α- and β-tocopherol on smooth muscle cell proliferation and protein kinase C activity. Quiescent cells are restimulated to grow with FCS (10%) in the presence of α-tocopherol and/or β-tocopherol (50 μ*M*). ***a*** After completion of the cell cycle (30 h) cells are counted with a hemocytometer. Viability is greater than 95%. Control (100%) represents $289 \pm 12 \times 103$ cells. ***b*** After 7 h restimulation, cells are permeabilized and protein kinase C is measured as described in Materials and Methods. Phorbol myristate acetate (100 n*M*) is added 60 min before assaying activity. The basal kinase activity is subtracted in all samples and only the PMA-stimulated activity is shown.

San Diego, Calif., USA. Other cell types such as Balb/3T3 mouse fibroblast and NB-2a mouse neuroblastoma are α-tocopherol-sensitive whereas CHO, Saos-2 human osteosarcoma cells, and P388 mouse macrophages are insensitive (table 1).

Effect of α-Tocopherol on Protein Kinase C Activity

The differential inhibition of protein kinase C by α-tocopherol and β-tocopherol is shown in figure 1B. As can be seen, β-tocopherol is much less effective and, as in the proliferation studies, prevents the inhibition of protein kinase C by α-tocopherol. The experiment reported in figure 2 shows that

Table 1. Antiproliferative effect of α-tocopherol is cell-specific

Tissue of origin	Sensitive	Insensitive
Rat aorta smooth muscle	A10/A7r5	
Human aorta smooth muscle	hAI	
Human Tenon's fibroblasts	hTF	
Human skin fibroblasts	CCD-SK	
Mouse neuroblastoma	NB2A	
Human pigmented		
Retinal epithelial cells	hPRE	
Human leukemia	U937	
Human prostate tumor	DU-145	
Mouse fibroblast	Balb/c-3T3	
Glioma	C6	
		Hela
Chinese hamster lung		LR73
Chinese hamster ovary		CHO
Human osteosarcoma		Saos-2
Mouse macrophage		P388 D1

Cells were made quiescent and restimulated with fetal calf serum in the presence or absence of α-tocopherol (50 μ*M*). Cells were counted after the completion of a cycle.

inhibition of protein kinase C and of proliferation occurs at the same range of α-tocopherol concentrations.

In the experiment shown in figure 3, the inhibition of protein kinase C activity by α-tocopherol has been studied as a function of the smooth muscle cell cycle. When α-tocopherol is added to G_0 cells, inhibition of protein kinase C activity is found when measured 7 h after fetal calf serum restimulation (fig. 3, inset). However, if α-tocopherol is added to G_1 cells and protein kinase C activity measured 7 h later, no inhibition is seen [17]. This result indicates that there is not direct interaction between α-tocopherol and protein kinase C and that α-tocopherol affects early events during the G_0/G_1 transition of the cell cycle. No changes at the level of transcription (not shown) or of protein kinase C expression during the G_1 phase in the absence or presence of α-tocopherol are observed (fig. 3) indicating that the oscillations of protein kinase C activity are the consequence of an alteration on the phosphorylation state of the enzyme. Related to this, α-tocopherol may act by inhibiting protein kinase C phosphorylation or stimulating its dephosphorylation (shown and discussed below).

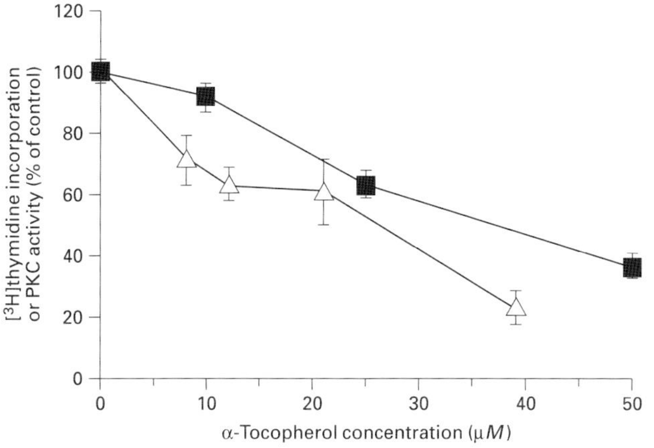

Fig. 2. Parallel inhibition of protein kinase C activity and of proliferation in smooth muscle cells. Quiescent cells are restimulated with FCS in the presence or absence of the indicated concentrations of α-tocopherol. After 7 h (cells in G_1-phase), protein kinase C is measured (■). Control (100%) corresponds to 138.6±4.9 pmol/min/106 cells. For DNA synthesis determination (△), [^{3}H]thymidine is given to the cells in the S-phase. Control represents 84,332±5,150 cpm. Results are expressed as mean±SD of triplicate determinations.

α-Tocopherol Inhibits Selectively Protein Kinase C-α

Gö 6976 at nanomolar concentrations inhibits protein kinase C-α and -βI, without affecting the other isoforms [18]. As can be seen in figure 4, when protein kinase C-α and -β are completely inhibited by Gö 6976, the residual activity is not sensitive to α-tocopherol indicating that the protein kinase C-δ, -ε, -ζ and -μ isoforms are not involved in the α-tocopherol-induced protein kinase C inhibition.

Taken together, the above experiments indicate that protein kinase C-α (and possibly -β) are the specific target for α-tocopherol action, a conclusion in complete agreement with the studies described below done by immunoprecipitating individual protein kinase C isoforms and measuring their activity.

Effect of α-Tocopherol on Protein Kinase C Isoforms Autophosphorylation

Autophosphorylation has been found to correlate with protein kinase C activity in immunoprecipitates. Cells are incubated in the absence or presence of α- or β-tocopherol for 7 h during the G_1 phase. Then, extracts are prepared and immunoprecipitation of the individual protein kinase C isoforms is performed. Cellular phosphorylation, autophosphorylation and histone phos-

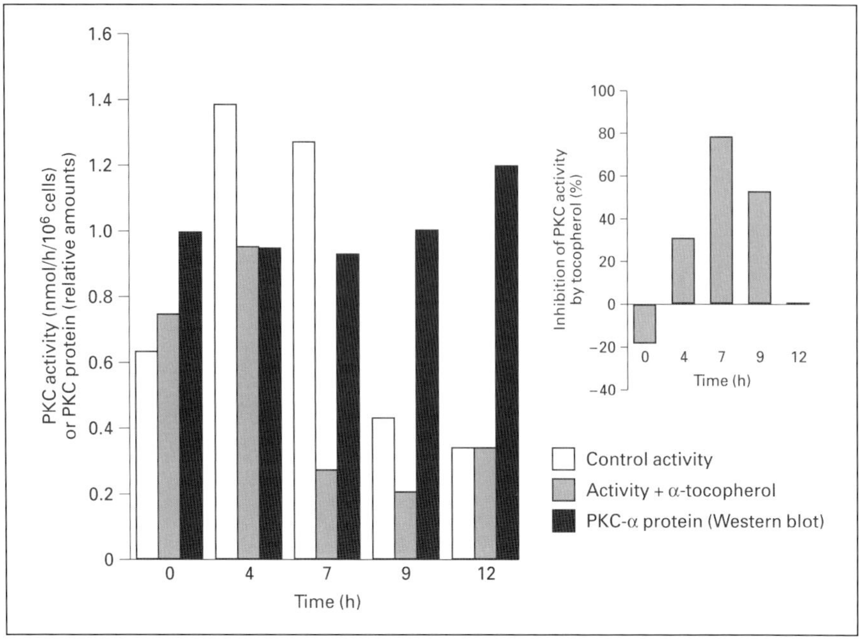

Fig. 3. Inhibition of protein kinase C activity by α-tocopherol is a function of the cycle. Qiescent cells (G_0) are stimulated for different times with FCS in the absence or presence of 50 μ*M* α-tocopherol. At the indicated points, PMA-stimulated protein kinase C activity is measured. Protein kinase C-α immunoblots are scanned by densitometry and signals are expressed as arbitrary units of absorbance.

phorylation are determined. As can be seen in table 2, protein kinase C-α from α-tocopherol-treated cells is inhibited. The activity of all other protein kinase C isoforms is not affected (not shown). On the other hand, β-tocopherol is without effect in all four protein kinase C isoforms studied.

Protein Phosphatase PP_2A Inhibition Abolishes the Effect of α-Tocopherol

When protein kinase C activity is measured in permeabilized cells in the presence of 2 n*M* okadaic acid (fig. 5) capable of inhibiting only protein phosphatase 2A (PP_2A), the effect of α-tocopherol disappears, showing that α-tocopherol affects the phosphorylation state of protein kinase C-α by changing the activity of PP_2A.

Effect of α-Tocopherol on Gene Expression

By differential display analysis it has been found that several genes of smooth muscle cells are differentially transcribed in the presence of α-tocoph-

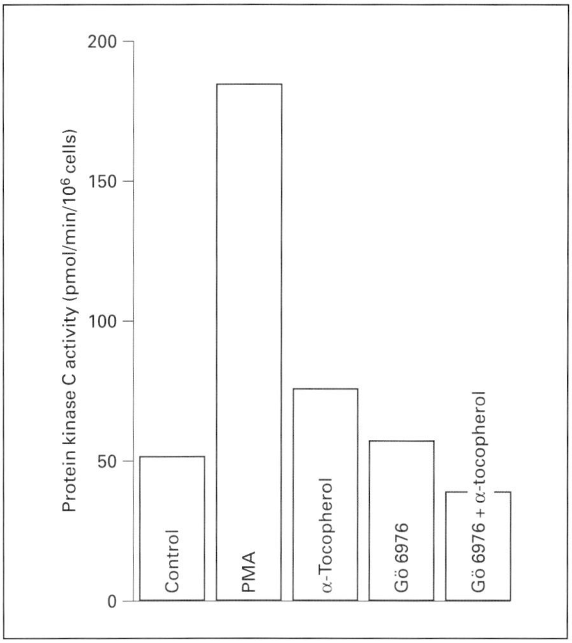

Fig. 4. Effect of α-tocoherol in the presence of protein kinase C-α inhibitors. Quiescent cells are restimulated for 7 h with FCS in the absence or presence of 50 μ*M* α-tocopherol. Gö 6976 (20 n*M*) was added to the permeabilized cells and protein kinase C is measured as described.

erol but not β-tocopherol. In particular, the gene of α-tropomyosin shows a transient enhancement of transcription as a function of the cell cycle time. α-Tropomyosin translation is also increased by α-tocopherol and not by β-tocopherol. Since no changes of mRNA stability can be observed in the presence of α-tocopherol, the data support the conclusion of a transcriptional control exerted by α-tocopherol on α-tropomyosin (data not shown).

Discussion

We have observed inhibition of smooth muscle cell proliferation in vitro by α-tocopherol at physiological concentrations. This could explain the notion that in vivo smooth muscle cells are quiescent and only multiply under stress conditions [19, 20]. Depletion of α-tocopherol, as a consequence of dietary or oxidative diminution, thus can lead to cell growth stimulation and develop-

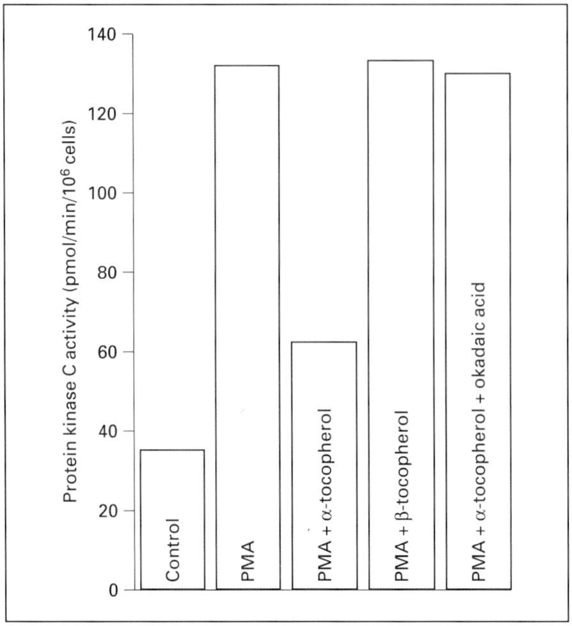

Fig. 5. Involvement of protein phosphatase 2A on the inhibition of protein kinase C by α-tocopherol. Cells are restimulated for 7 h with FCS in the presence or absence of 50 μ*M* α- or β-tocopherol. Okadaic acid (2 n*M*) is added 1 h before the protein kinase C assay. Values are determined using the phosphatase-insensitive peptide $MBP_{(4-14)}$ as a substrate.

ment of atherosclerosis. β-Tocopherol, an antioxidant almost as potent as α-tocopherol, does not show any effect at the level of cell proliferation or protein kinase C activity. Since β-tocopherol prevents and does not potentiate the effects of α-tocopherol, it appears justifiable to conclude that the mechanism of action of α-tocopherol as a regulator of smooth muscle cell proliferation cannot be associated with its antioxidant properties. Moreover, the above results can be the consequence of the existence of a common intermediate, a putative α-tocopherol-binding protein, that should bind α- and β-tocopherol at the same site, α-tocopherol acting as an agonist and β-tocopherol as an antagonist.

Protein kinase C inhibition appears to be necessary to cause smooth muscle cell proliferation inhibition in vitro but how this enzyme is inhibited by α-tocopherol is not fully clarified. A direct interaction of α-tocopherol with protein kinase C has been excluded on the basis of the cell cycle dependence and cell type specificity. Moreover, no changes in the expression of the protein in the presence of α-tocopherol has been observed. By using isoform-specific

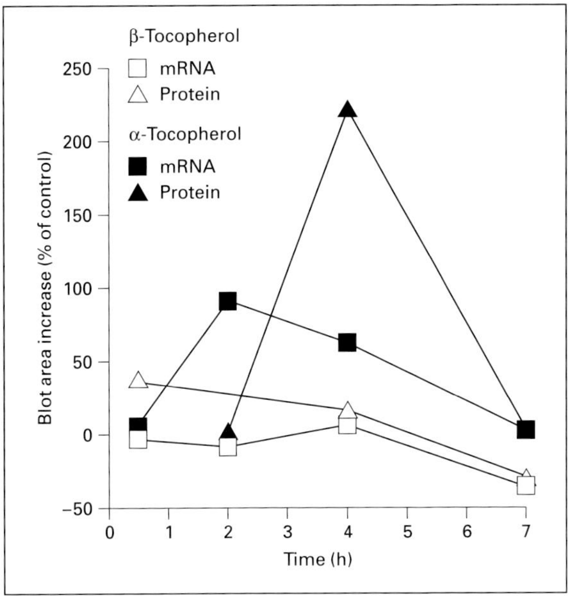

Fig. 6. Effect of α-tocopherol on gene expression. Cells are restimulated for 7 h with FCS in the presence or absence of 50 μ*M* α- or β-tocopherol. From cell extracts at different incubation times, Northern and Western blots are made using an exon 12 α-tropomyosin probe and antibodies against human α-tropomyosin.

inhibitors and activators (Gö 6976 and C_2-ceramide) it is found that the protein kinase C-α isoform is the target of α-tocopherol action.

It is known that protein kinase C becomes active as a consequence of a permissive phosphorylation and an autophosphorylation at discrete sites [21, 22]. Thus, a lack of phosphorylation of protein kinase C by α-tocopherol may be involved in its inhibitory effects. By incubating smooth muscle cell with $^{32}P_i$ it is found that protein kinase C-α phosphorylation is strongly diminished by α-tocopherol. To address further this question, the autophosphorylation activity of individual immunoprecipitated protein kinase C isoforms has been studied. A specific inhibition by α-tocopherol in the autophosphorylation of protein kinase C-α but not in the other protein kinase C isoforms is found.

Accordingly, the following scenario can be imagined: in the presence of α-tocopherol and during the transition $G_0 \rightarrow G_1$, an inhibition of protein kinase C-α phosphorylation or activation of its dephosphorylation occurs. This posttranslational change results in a less active enzyme. The effect of α-tocopherol disappears when the cells are treated with okadaic acid,

Table 2. Effect of α- and β-tocopherol on protein kinase C-α phosphorylation state, autophosphorylating activity and activity towards histone III-S

	^{32}P-protein kinase C-α %	Autophosphorylating activity of protein kinase C-α, %	Histone activity %
PMA	100	100	100
α-Tocopherol	18.5	36.4	56.0
β-Tocopherol	74.1	84.9	79.0

Quiescent A7r5 cells were incubated in phosphate-free medium for 48 h. Cells received 0.25 mCi/ml ^{32}Pi for the last 14 h. Cells were restimulated for 7 h with fetal calf serum in the presence of 50 μ*M* α-tocopherol or β-tocopherol. PMA (100 n*M*) was added for the last hour as indicated. Cell extracts were prepared and proteins resolved by SDS-PAGE. For activity, after treatment of cells, extracts were prepared, protein kinase C-α was immunoprecipitated and kinase reactions in the absence (autophosphorylation) or presence (kinase activity) of histone III-S were performed. Proteins were resolved in a 10% SDS-PAGE and radioactive bands were quantified with a BioRad Molecular-Analyst software. Protein amount was estimated by staining the gel with the SYPRO kit or by immunoblots with the MC5 antibody. Data are expressed as percent of maximal protein kinase C phosphorylation or activity obtained in the presence of PMA alone.

suggesting that the inhibition of protein kinase C phosphorylation may occur by activation of a phosphatase of the 2A type. Indeed the activity of this phosphatase is increased in vitro by α-tocopherol. The question remains open as to the mechanism of α-tocopherol activation of PP_2A. Studies in progress will clarify if in the G_0 to G_1 transition, activation of a pre-existing phosphatase or its new expression is caused by the presence of α-tocopherol.

In conclusion, the specificity of α-tocopherol effects are indicative of a site-directed recognition mechanism and at physiological concentrations the following events may take place: binding of α-tocopherol to a 'receptor protein', activation (or expression) of a protein phosphatase (PP_2A), dephosphorylation of protein kinase C resulting in its inhibition, effects at the level of gene transcription such as the transient increase in α-tropomyosin, followed by final inhibition of cell proliferation. On the other side, if the amount of cellular α-tocopherol content is too low, due to diet, malabsorption or high oxidative stress, the above sequence of events may result into a high level of cell proliferation.

Finally, the epidemiological information linking a decrease of plasma α-tocopherol with an increased risk of ischemic heart disease finds in these studies a molecular counterpart.

Acknowledgment

The present study has been supported by the Swiss National Science Foundation and by F. Hoffmann-La Roche, AG.

References

1 Vieira AV, Schneider WJ, Vieira PM: Retinoids: Transport, metabolism, and mechanisms of action. J Endocrinol 1995;146:201–207.

2 Ng, KW, Zhou H, Manji S, Martin TJ: Regulation and regulatory role of the retinoids. Crit Rev Eukaryot Gene Expr 1995;5:219–253.

3 Fisher GJ, Voorhees JJ: Molecular mechanisms of retinoid actions in skin. FASEB J 1996;10: 1002–1013.

4 Love, JM, Gudas LJ: Vitamin A, differentiation and cancer. Curr Opin Cell Biol 1994;6:825–831.

5 Harada H, Miki R, Masushige S, Kato S: Gene expression of retinoic acid receptors, retinoid-X receptors, and cellular retinol-binding protein I in bone and its regulation by vitamin A. Endocrinology 1995;136:5329–5355.

6 White JA, Guo YD, Baetz K, Beckett Jones B, Bonasoro J, Hsu KE, Dilworth FJ, Jones G, Petkovich M: Identification of the retinoic acid-inducible *all-trans*-retinoic acid 4-hydroxylase. J Biol Chem 1996;271:29922–29927.

7 Pan L, Eckhoff C, Brinckerhoff CE: Suppression of collagenase gene expression by *all-trans-* and 9-*cis*-retinoic acid is ligand-dependent and requires both RARs and RXRs. J Cell Biochem 1995; 57:575–589.

8 Bertram JS: Inhibition of chemically induced neoplastic transformation by carotenoids. Mechanistic studies. Ann NY Acad Sci 1993;686:161–175.

9 Zhang LX, Cooney RV, Bertram JS: Carotenoids up-regulate connexin43 gene expression independent of their provitamin A or antioxidant properties. Cancer Res 1992;52:5707–5712.

10 Mahmoodian F, Gosiewska A, Peterkofsky B: Regulation and properties of bone alkaline phosphatase during vitamin C deficiency in guinea pigs. Arch Biochem Biophys 1996;336:86–96.

11 Wang XT, Culotta VC, Klee CB: Superoxide dismutase protects calcineurin from inactivation. Nature 1996;383:434–437.

12 Klee CB, Wang X: Coupling between oxidative stress and calcium signaling. FASEB J 1997;11: A1120.

13 Christakos S, Raval Pandya M, Wernyj RP, Yang W: Genomic mechanisms involved in the pleiotropic actions of 1,25-dihdroxyvitamin D3 [erratum appears in Biochem J 1996;318:1079]. Biochem J 1996;316: 361–371.

14 Nishikawa Y, Carr BI, Wang M, Kar S, Finn F, Dowd P, Zheng ZB, Kerns J, Naganathan S: Growth inhibition of hepatoma cells induced by vitamin K and its analogs. J Biol Chem 1995;270: 28304–28310.

15 Wang Z, Wang M, Finn F, Car BI: The growth inhibitory effects of vitamins K and their actions on gene expression. Hepatology 1995;22:876–882.

16 Azzi A, Boscoboinik D, Marilley D, Özer NK, Stäuble B, Tasinato A: Vitamin E: A sensor and an information transducer of the cell oxidation state. Am J Clin Nutr 1995;62(suppl):1337–1346.

17 Tasinato A, Boscoboinik D, Bartoli GM, Maroni P, Azzi A: *d*-α-Tocopherol inhibition of vascular smooth muscle cell proliferation occurs at physiological concentrations, correlates with protein kinase C inhibition, and is independent of its antioxidant properties. Proc Natl Acad Sci USA 1995;92:12190–12194.

18 Martiny Baron G, Kazanietz MG, Mischak H, Blumberg PM, Kochs G, Hug H, Marme D, Schachtele C: Selective inhibition of protein kinase C isozymes by the indolocarbazole Gö 6976. J Biol Chem 1993;268:9194–9197.

19 Raines EW, Ross R: Smooth muscle cells and the pathogenesis of the lesions of atherosclerosis. Br Heart J 1993;69:S30–S37.
20 Clowes AW, Schwartz SM: Significance of quiescent smooth muscle migration in the injured rat carotid artery. Circ Res 1985;56:139–145.
21 Newton AC: Protein kinase C: Structure, function, and regulation. J Biol Chem 1995;270:28495–28498.
22 Dutil EM, Keranen LM, DePaoli-Roach AA, Newton AC: In vivo regulation of protein kinase C by trans-phosphorylation followed by autophosphorylation. J Biol Chem 1994;269:29359–29362.

Prof. A. Azzi, University of Bern, Institute of Biochemicals & Molecular Biology,
Brühlstrasse 28, CH–3012 Bern (Switzerland)
Tel. +41 31 631 4131, Fax +41 31 631 3737, E-Mail azzi@mci.unibe.ch

Walter P, Hornig D, Moser U (eds): Functions of Vitamins beyond Recommended Dietary Allowances. Bibl Nutr Dieta. Basel, Karger, 2001, No 55, pp 189–191

Folic Acid, Vitamins B_6 and B_{12}: Relation to Homocysteine and Cardiovascular Disease

F.J. Kok

Department of Epidemiology and Public Health, Wageningen, The Netherlands

Evidence for Recommendation

Epidemiological studies and experimental data strongly suggest that plasma total homocysteine (tHcy) is a risk factor for CVD. So far, results from prospective studies show less strong risk estimates as compared to those of case-control studies. Moreover, since controlled intervention trials are lacking it is still unclear whether the association is causal.

The association is, as for serum cholesterol, graded, i.e. CVD risk is steadily increasing with increasing levels of tHcy. From the shape of the risk curve it can be estimated that each 10% increase in tHcy is associated with approximately 15% increase in CVD risk. This suggests quite a strong impact of tHcy if we compare these figures with those of total cholesterol (30% risk increase for each 10% increase in cholesterol). Lowering tHcy plasma concentration may therefore be beneficial. According to the risk curve, it would be desirable to establish a tHcy level as low as possible. Although adverse effects have not been observed in subjects who achieved very low levels, more detailed research is necessary. From the available data it seems that tHcy levels <7 µmol/l are difficult to reach. Although 7 µmol/l is achievable, it is not necessarily optimal. There is quite some variability in plasma tHcy levels. In healthy blood donors ranges from 7.9 to 9.3 µmol/l have been observed. Hyperhomocysteinemia is defined as plasma levels >16.3 µmol/l.

Intervention studies have revealed that folic acid is the major determinant of tHcy. In combination with folic acid, vitamins B_6 and B_{12} may have some additional beneficial effect on tHcy. The most recent intervention studies have shown that 200 μg/day of folic acid supplements on top of usual dietary folate intake is most effective in reducing tHcy. Subjects with higher baseline tHcy levels seem to benefit more from extra folic acid than those with lower initial levels. Expressed in dietary folate intake, taking into account bioavailability, this would imply that at least 500 μg/day of dietary folate would be required for optimal tHcy levels. Observational studies in which the folate intake was plotted against plasma tHcy levels, found that tHcy levels reached its nadir at dietary folate intakes of 350–400 μg/day and higher.

The recommended daily allowances (RDA) are folic acid 200–300 μg/day, for vitamin B_6 1–1.5 mg/day, and for vitamin B_{12} 1–2 μg/day. In the working group session it was concluded that there is not sufficient evidence for definite recommendations at or beyond the RDAs. The current mean dietary folate intake for adults in Europe is for males 291 μg/day (range 197–326) and for females 247/μg/day (range 168–320).

Missing Scientific Knowledge

To prove causality trial data are urgently needed. A few randomized controlled trials of the type of secondary prevention using hard endpoints (CVD recurrence and mortality) have recently been started in Oxford (UK) and Boston (USA). However, primary prevention trials are much more needed. One such trial using an intermediate endpoint (carotid artery wall thickening) was started at the beginning of 1998 in Wageningen (The Netherlands).

Controlled dietary intervention studies should identify the optimal dose of folic acid/dietary folate to decrease plasma tHcy. So far, 200 μg/day of extra folic acid has shown to be effective, however, a lower dose may be sufficient as well. Since the bioavailability of folate in foods is only 50–70% because of the high amount of polyglutamate as compared to monoglutamate, it is important to find ways (e.g. new techniques in food processing) to increase the mono/polyglutamate ratio. These foods and other (fortified) foods need to be evaluated on their potential to lower tHcy. Further insight in the genetic risk associated with polymorphisms such as 5,10-methylenetetrahydrofolate reductase (MTHFR) and the interaction with folate is needed. Current data indicate that MTHFR polymorphism is not associated strongly with risk of CVD. It has been suggested that only in subjects who combine the genotype with low folate intake, the risk is increased. Finally, research on plausible biological mechanisms is necessary to shed light on the pathophysiology of homocysteine and CVD.

Time Scale

The members of the working group estimated a period of about 5 years before the issue of folate-tHcy-CVD would have developed in a way that more definite recommendations could be formulated.

Communication to Consumers

General advice to the public at large to consume more fruits and vegetables is recommended. A total of at least 400 g/day of fruits and vegetables (5–7 servings daily) would help to increase the folate intake to the desired level of 350 μg/day or more. Individuals with high (genetic) risk may be advised to take a supplement daily containing 200 μg of folic acid in addition to a diet rich in fruits and vegetables.

Prof. F. Kok, Department of Epidemiology and Public Health,
P.O. Box 238, NL–6700 AE Wageningen (The Netherlands)
Tel. +31 8370 82580/82080, Fax +31 3174 82782, E-Mail frans.kok@medew.hegl.wau.nl

Walter P, Hornig D, Moser U (eds): Functions of Vitamins beyond Recommended Dietary Allowances. Bibl Nutr Dieta. Basel, Karger, 2001, No 55, pp 192–195

Evidence of Folic Acid and Folate in the Prevention of Neural Tube Defects

J.M. Scott

Biochemistry Department, Trinity College, University of Dublin, Ireland

The neural plate closes to form the neural tube beginning at day 21 postconception and ending at day 27, resulting in the formation of what will eventually be the spinal column. At the same time a protrusion extends to encompass the cranium. Incomplete closure of the former structure results in a spinal cord with an opening in it and produces the condition known as spina bifida. The outcome varies from being very minor, through a spectrum of disabilities where the child will have paralysis of lower limbs and bladder often accompanied by hydrocephalus because of impaired drainage of cerebrospinal fluid from the brain. Incomplete closure of the cranium is called anencephaly and is incompatible with life with the embryo dying either in the uterus or shortly after birth. Both conditions are called neural tube defects (NTDs). Historically the prevalence of NTDs varied from country to country with communities of Celtic origin having a particularly high prevalence. The prevalence at its height in such communities was often as high as 6/1,000 births. It has reduced in most communities to values of less than 2/1,000. While much of this is due in many communities to early diagnosis and termination, there is general agreement that the prevalence has dropped in most communities independent of such intervention. Despite these reductions, NTDs represent the most common congenital birth defect. It has long been recognized that NTDs arise from a genetic predisposition interacting with an environmental factor, probably a nutrient or nutrients. It is now accepted by all experts in this field that this nutrient is the vitamin folate. It has been shown conclusively that the synthetic form of this vitamin (folic acid) prevents the majority of NTDs if taken preconceptionally by women before the closure of the neural tube. The evidence for this is that various types of intervention trials with folic acid have shown a dramatic reduction of NTDs. It is also backed up by a large number of case-control studies. Most of these studies used 400 μg of the synthetic form of the vitamin folic acid because that was the form and the amount that existed in supplements used in the trials and case-control studies.

As a result of the above studies, the UK Department of Health and the CDC in Atlanta came out with recommendations that women should take an extra 400 μg/day of folic acid/folate to prevent NTDs. This recommendation was subsequently adopted by many other countries. It meant that a level of folic acid higher than the RDA was being recommended to a large sector of healthy people, because the RDA in most centres is 200 μg or less. It was suggested that this advice could be acted upon by individual women by (a) increasing their intake of food folate, (b) taking folic acid-fortified foods currently available in many but not all countries, and (c) taking supplements (tablets) containing folic acid. It was agreed at the workshop that while it may be possible for a woman to obtain some protection from an NTD-affected birth by increasing her intake of a food folate (a) it would be very difficult in practice to get optimum protection. This is for three reasons: Firstly, there is no single food (apart from liver that potentially pregnant women are advised not to take) that has a high concentration of folate. Secondly, unlike the synthetic form of the vitamin folic acid, shown to be effective in the intervention trials and case-control studies, natural folate is conjugated to a long polyglutamyl chain and must be deconjugated in the intestine prior to its absorption. This consequently reduces its bioavailability perhaps by as much as half. Finally, while synthetic folic acid is chemically quite stable, reduction of the pteridine ring as occurs in natural folates renders them chemically very unstable, resulting in considerable loss during harvesting storage and preparation. Supplements (b) at the level of 400 μg/day have shown to be effective in the trials. They will of course offer an ideal form of protection. The problem here is with compliance. In most communities over half of pregnancies are unplanned. In addition, to get the information across to those who plan pregnancies that folic acid is protective in preventing these important birth defects has proved difficult. Finally, even if women have this information there are some who still fail to comply with the advice on a regular basis. The lack of success with these two options (a and b) has led most regulatory agencies to consider mandatory fortification (c). One such agency, i.e. the FDA in the USA, has adopted mandatory fortification of a staple in the diet, namely flour. While such mandatory fortification could be arranged to ensure that all would receive optimum levels of folic acid through this measure, the problem is that to do so would involve putting sufficient folic acid to achieve the target dose of 400 μg in very small amounts of flour. This is because those on low intake of flour would need 400 μg in a small amount. This would of necessity mean that those women and more importantly members of the population as a whole who ingested large amounts of flour products would get perhaps over 1.0 mg/day. These higher amounts are a concern because they are known to treat the anaemia in the vitamin B_{12} malabsorption condition called pernicious anaemia (PA). This phenomenon, often called the making of the anaemia as suggested, will prevent the early diagnosis of the condition in some patients allowing the neuropathy also associated with this condition to progress undiagnosed to a point where it may be partially irreversible. It is felt by some that PA is extremely rare and is now always diagnosed at the early stages of the neuropathy. There is good reason to believe that this is the case but still this concern specifically about PA but also of other possible unknown effects of continuous exposure to high levels of folic acid has resulted in a pressure to try to ensure that sectors of the general public are not exposed to large daily intakes of folic acid. Consequently, the FDA adopted a level of fortification that would increase the average rate of folic acid in the US diet by 100 μg/day. While this falls short of the target of 400 μg/day, there is reason to believe that it may have a disproportional benefit. This is because the risk of NTD may be very high in those with the lowest intakes. It could thus be expected that even a small increase would move such women to a better albeit not optimal status with respect to folate.

The consensus reached in the working group was that while improvement in intake of natural folates may help, it will be difficult and far from optimal. There are two alternatives open to any community. Continue to try to improve the taking of supplements. Alternatively, a community might decide to fortify the diet. In the latter instance because of concerns about overexposure in the elderly and other sectors it is unlikely that currently accepted target levels to prevent NTDs (i.e. 400 μg/day) will be sought. Perhaps in that circumstance a policy of fortification to what may be recognized as a suboptimal level could be undertaken (say 100 μg/day) in parallel with continued efforts to get women of childbearing age to take supplements. This policy would have benefits for the more disadvantaged by a positive improvement in their diet. It would also continue to strive to achieve optimum protection by informing everybody of the necessity to take supplements. The combination of the two where it was done would achieve optimal protection without any significant increase in risk. This is because the two levels together are unlikely to reach levels that will mask PA. In addition, women of childbearing age are at a very low risk of having PA. One would have to weigh this very low risk against the certain benefit of folic acid in preventing NTD.

Missing Knowledge and Time Taken to Rectify

(1) Determination of lower levels of folic acid that may be effective in preventing NTDs. While new intervention trials at lower doses are not possible, one should be able to demonstrate a relationship between folate status and risk of an NTD. Time frame – immediate.

(2) At the levels that are likely to be used for fortification, potential hazards are considered to be extremely unlikely. However, thought should be given to how to recognize such hazards if they were to occur. Time frame – ongoing.

(3) NTDs are known to be an interplay of a nutrient now known to folic acid/folate with a genetic predisposition. One genetic variant involved has been identified (the 5,10-methylenetetrahydrofolate reductase thermoliable variant). It however only accounts for some 13% of NTDs. Since over three-quarters of NTDs are probably preventable by folic acid/folate, there are some 60% variants to be discovered. Time frame to identify new variants – 2–5 years.

Communication to the Public

(1) In communities not planning mandatory fortification to continue to encourage women who may become pregnant to take supplements.

(2) In communities who may use fortified food to begin a debate on the benefits. If low levels are used for fortification to recognize that while this will not give optimum protection and that consequently there is a continued need for women to take supplements. If high levels of fortification are used it will be necessary to educate healthcare professionals of possible risks associated with fortification even though such risks may be small.

Prof. John Scott, University of Dublin, Trinity College,
Biochemistry Department, Dublin 2 (Ireland)
Tel. +35 3608 1974, Fax +35 1677 2400, E-Mail jscott@tcd.ie

Walter P, Hornig D, Moser U (eds): Functions of Vitamins beyond Recommended Dietary Allowances. Bibl Nutr Dieta. Basel, Karger, 2001, No 55, pp 196–199

Functions of Antioxidant Vitamins beyond RDAs

A.T. Diplock[†], *G. van Poppel*

Occupational Toxicology and Nutrition, TNO Nutrition and Food Research Institute, Zeist, The Netherlands

The hypothesis that antioxidants may lower the risk of certain degenerative diseases was considered to be very plausible. However, the evidence available at present was insufficient for a definite recommendation to be made that the human intake of any antioxidant should be increased to a level beyond the Recommended Dietary Allowance (RDA). There was in particular persuasive evidence that some benefit could be obtained by increasing the intake of vitamin E to a level above that which could be obtained through manipulation of normal dietary constituents, but long-term safety considerations require that caution should be exercised in this regard. Despite the availability of considerable evidence that vitamin E is safe at levels of intake up to at least 1,000 times the RDA, these trials were conducted over rather short periods of time. There is no conclusive evidence that such a high level of vitamin E when consumed for long periods of time is entirely safe and free from undesirable side effects.

In order to answer the outstanding questions concerning the health benefit that might be derived from increased levels of intake of antioxidants above the RDA, there are four general areas in which data is incomplete or missing. These are as follows: (i) Clinical trials are required, particularly of the interventional kind, to establish whether addition to the diet of antioxidants beyond the RDA level may have an effect in reducing the risk of disease. Although the ultimate test of this hypothesis is the lowering of the risk of an identified disease itself, carefully chosen early markers for that disease endpoint can be expected to provide evidence more quickly, because the natural history of human degenerative diseases is very long, which increases the cost of trials to a prohibitive level and does not meet the urgent need for answers to these questions in the shortest possible time. (ii) Markers (sometimes called biomarkers); there are several markers available which purport to provide indicators of the consequences of free radical damage to human cellular components. These require validation in at least three ways: (a) intra-laboratory study of the variability of the measures obtained using identical biological material; (b) similar studies between a number of different laboratories in different parts of the world, using apparently identical methods and carrying out the assays on identical material which has been produced and distributed from a common centre; (c) the question of the relevance of a selected marker to a genuine human tissue disorder, which may lead to disease, and the relevance of antioxidant protection in this. The marker must be genuinely relevant to an eventual disease which is the paradigm for the putative risk-lowering function of an antioxidant. (iii) Studies of the bioavailability of the antioxidants are urgently required. Much of the available evidence comes from animal studies and there is little reliable evidence of a truly human kind which explores the question of the uptake, distribution and tissue concentration of antioxidants. (iv) There are a number of remaining questions regarding the safety of antioxidants. Thus the safety of long-term exposure to antioxidants at high levels of intake has not been examined, and the question of exposure to antioxidants at supranormal levels of intake, in special population groups, such as heavy smokers and heavy drinkers of alcohol, needs urgent careful study.

The question was examined of the timescale for obtaining results from the studies suggested above. Although opinions varied somewhat, it was agreed that up to 10 years were needed for the results of clinical trials using short-term endpoints, and that up to 30 years would probably be required for more detailed studies involving functional markers linked to an identifiable ultimate disease. The resolution of the remaining questions about the validation of markers would be achieved quite quickly, and would have to precede the clinical studies so that the timeframe suggested would include time for these developments.

There was detailed discussion on the concept of communication of research findings to the consumer in the antioxidant area and on the impact that this might be expected to have on public health. The purpose of such communication is to identify guidelines which might be established, and more general information which need not be of the same stringency. Scientific organizations have a role to play in receiving and discussing such information, and being responsible for the dissemination of research findings to other professionals and to the public, i.e. the consumer. It was generally agreed that it is in the nature of science that there would be disagreement among scientists about the detailed conclusions to be arrived at. However, there was a strong recommendation that such disagreement should not be allowed to prevent the dissemination of useful health advice to the public and that scientists have a moral duty to be at the forefront of providing useful information, even though there might not be complete agreement within the scientific community as to the detail of what might be regarded as established fact. Using a strictly scientific approach, it was agreed that no recommendations could be made to enhance the level of intake of antioxidants above the RDA, and in this discussion it was importantly emphasized that another vital priority was to emphasize to the public the need to achieve RDA amounts of certain nutrients in their daily diet; there is extensive evidence that in many parts of the world, including USA, UK and other European countries, the level of intake of certain nutrients has fallen below the RDA. In the antioxidant context, the recommendation to take between 5 and 7 servings of fruit and vegetables per day was agreed as the primary advice to be given and consideration of increasing the intake above the RDA must be in relation to this general advice. In this respect, it was considered that not only the nutrient antioxidants vitamins C and E, and carotenoids, but also nonnutrients such as polyphenols, may be of importance. Considerations of safety are paramount in increasing antioxidant intake, and recent findings with respect to β-carotene supplements in heavy habitual smokers have led to concern and the need for caution in recommending high intakes of this nutrient which, until the advent of these studies, was considered entirely safe even at a high level of intake. In view of the conviction of the majority of the members of the Working Group that the scientific community have a moral duty to give advice in the area of antioxidant intake, consideration was given to the question of what might be communicated to the public about this question. An important consideration was that, on the one hand, any statement should not raise false expectations as to the likely benefits of antioxidants, and on the other hand that the statement should not be so negative as to fail to reflect the considerable evidence that does exist with regard to the health benefits of antioxidants. Bearing these considerations in mind, the following points were agreed as being an accurate statement of the present position: (i) That it is a plausible hypothesis that increased intakes of antioxidants may confer health benefits with respect to degenerative diseases, particularly cardiovascular disease and some forms of cancer. (ii) That the consumers should in the first instance make sure that their diet contains sufficient essential nutrients that the RDAs of all of them are achieved. (iii) That 5–7 servings of fruits and vegetables in the diet are agreed to be beneficial in reducing the risk of cancer in some body sites, and of cardiovascular disease. (iv) Increasing the intake of antioxidants beyond the RDA amounts may have some health benefits; the risks are probably small but some adverse effects cannot yet be excluded. Particular regard must be had to special groups such as heavy smokers, and heavy drinkers of alcohol, where adverse effects may be a problem. (v) In general, the intake of extra antioxidants is safe as long as it does not exceed the level of intake to be expected from 5–7 servings of fruits and vegetables. A special case can be made for vitamin E where ingestion of up to 200 mg/day may be beneficial in reducing the risk of cardiovascular disease, but long-term safety considerations cannot be excluded.

Dr. Geert van Poppel, Occupational Toxicology and Nutrition,
TNO Nutrition and Food Research Institute, P.O. Box 360,
NL-3700 AJ Zeist (The Netherlands)
Fax +31 30 694 49 28

Walter P, Hornig D, Moser U (eds): Functions of Vitamins beyond Recommended Dietary Allowances. Bibl Nutr Dieta. Basel, Karger, 2001, No 55, pp 200–205

Vitamins and Immunocompetence

Jeffrey B. Blumberg[a], *David A. Hughes*[b]

[a] USDA Human Nutrition Research Center on Aging, Tufts University, Boston, Mass., USA; and
[b] Nutrition, Diet & Health Department, Institute of Food Research, Norwich Laboratory, Norwich, UK

In his seminal work more than 50 years ago, Axelrod stated that 'in the study of nutrition, any measure of animal performance can be utilized for the evaluation of diets. Antibody production, the normal physiological response to an antigenic stimulus, might be expected to provide a measure of nutritional status...'. Later, Scrimshaw et al. [1959] critically analyzed the body of available scientific information and detailed the interactions between nutrition and infection; they incepted a new period of research by offering that 'the idea that nutritional deficiencies and infections have something to do with each other follows from the historical association between famine and pestilence. Numerous field and clinical observations and many experimental studies support this view.' It is now well established that nutritional status can have a profound impact on the immune system, in part because so many measures of immune function can be readily assessed [Gershwin et al., 1985; Chandra, 1992]. Thus, it seems opportune now to raise four key questions regarding the status of the field.

1. Do we have sufficient evidence to make recommendations for increasing the current allowance of vitamins to beneficially affect immune function?

Anderson [1995, 2000] has reviewed the influence of vitamins on human immune function. It appears clear that most research studies have been conducted in populations with marked vitamin deficiencies or in the elderly. However, many nutritional deficiencies can be complicated by infections [Keusch and Farthing, 1986] which affect both vitamin status and immune function. The elderly have been characterized as generally presenting with a poor nutritional status and age-related impairments in immune responsiveness [Blumberg, 1996]. Thus, extrapolating the results from these studies to dietary recommendations for generally healthy adults may not be entirely valid. Studies examining the effect of vitamins at doses approximating commonly recommended intakes for healthy young children and adults are rare. Indeed, such studies present a challenge as 'optimal' immune responsiveness is measured against standard values typical of healthy young adults. It is not clear that increasing immune functions beyond this level is desirable.

Concern has been expressed about the potential for adverse effects upon immune function from supra-dietary vitamin intakes. For example, the failure to find a chemopreventive effect of β-carotene within three major prospective trials [Alpha-Tocopherol, Beta-Carotene Cancer Prevention Study Group 1994; Omenn et al., 1996; Hennekens et al., 1996] using supplementation of ≥25 mg/day indicates no benefit and some potential for harm in heavy chronic smokers. However, a test of immune function carried out within the Physicians' Health Study suggests that high-dose β-carotene may nonetheless have a beneficial effect on natural killer cell activity, a function relevant to cancer prevention, particularly in the elderly [Santos et al., 1996]. β-Carotene supplementation also appears to enhance tumor surveillance in nonsmoking middle-aged volunteers [Hughes et al., 1997] and increase the frequency of helper/inducer T lymphocytes in healthy adults [Alexander et al., 1985].

It is worthwhile noting that vitamin requirements for optimal immunity may vary based upon specific dietary patterns. For example, diets rich in polyunsaturated fatty acids, which are more prone to oxidative damage than saturated fatty acids, appear to require a higher intake of antioxidant vitamins such as vitamin E. These types of nutrient-nutrient interactions impacting on immune function may limit the ability to make broad recommendations regarding optimal vitamin intakes for populations with differing dietary habits.

While it appears premature at this time to offer specific recommendations for vitamin intake to the general population, the evidence of a boosting effect by vitamins on immune function in the elderly suggests that increasing the intakes, especially of the antioxidant vitamins, might be beneficial [Meydani et al., 1995; Chandra, 1997]. However, optimal daily intakes remain undetermined.

2. What knowledge must be obtained before new vitamin recommendations for optimal immunity can be developed?

Since the first studies in nutritional immunology 50 years ago, our greater understanding now of the complexity of the immune system has allowed for experimental assessment of each of its constituent parts, e.g., in peripheral blood, lymph nodes, spleen, thymus, tonsils, bone marrow, etc. [Beisel 1992a, b]. This is an important issue as the microenvironment of each of these elements of the immune system may be differentially responsive to specific nutrients [Cunningham-Rundles, 1993]. However, many of these tissues are

Table 1. Measure of human immune function: global assessment in vivo

Noninvasive	Invasive
Antibiotic use	Antibody titers to vaccines, acute-phase proteins
Fever duration	Delayed-type hypersensitivity skin test response
Hospitalization duration	Immune cell/receptor subsets
Infection rate	Virus concentrations in serum and other bodily fluids
Severity of infection	

Table 2. Measures of human immune function: cellular assessment in vitro

Cytotoxicity by natural killer cells and T cells
Immune cell mediators: interleukins, interferons, immunoglobulins and other cytokines
Phagocytosis by neutrophils and macrophages
Proliferation stimulated by mitogens or antigens

only available in studies of animal models. Nonetheless, there are a number of practical methods for the clinical assessment of immune responsiveness [Bendich, 1995].

In vivo tests represent the most reliable determination of immune function as in vitro measures cannot reflect the full array of physiologic and metabolic influences which impact immune responses. Nonetheless, in vitro assays are an important research tool. They can help provide some insight into the mechanisms and specificity of action, and reveal the potential for subtle effects masked in in vivo situations. Commonly employed measures of in vivo and in vitro human immune function are listed in tables 1 and 2. In clinical trials, leukocytic profiles of peripheral blood, readily assessed by fluorescence-activated cell sorter, provide immediate insight into the potential for alterations in the proportion and number of circulating immune cells and suggest the array of in vitro tests to be performed. The increasing sophistication of analytical techniques, e.g., the ability to distinguish between different T-helper cell subpopulations by their cytokine-producting profiles [Mosmann and Sad, 1996], now allow for the exploration of very subtle influences by vitamins on the immune system in healthy individuals. Antibody responses, measured by ELISA or radioimmunoassay, to vaccinations are an excellent functional test of humoral-mediated immunity. Delayed-type hypersensitivity cutaneous responses are a practical, if semiquantitative, measure of T-mediated cellular immunity although consideration must be given to confounding by recall or booster effects. Noninvasive proxy measures of immunity such as the duration of fever or antibiotic use should not be overlooked as meaningful tests, particularly in the context of a well-controlled trial, as they are also relevant to considerations of healthcare cost-benefit ratios.

In considering the outcome of research studies, it is worthwhile to consider the relevant endpoints. The impact of vitamin deficiency on immunocompetence is recognized and it appears as though generally recommended dietary intakes are sufficient to prevent significant impairments in function such as anergy. However, it is not clear that these intakes are optimized for levels of immune function associated with a reduced risk of infectious diseases, noninfectious inflammatory conditions, cancer or mortality, particularly in certain populations such as the elderly. Indeed, these endpoints are rarely measured in clinical trials studying the effect of vitamins on immunocompetence.

3. How long will it take to obtain the missing knowledge?

Although the work has yet to be undertaken, a large amount of useful information on the relationship between vitamin intake and optimal immunity could be obtained in a relatively short timeframe, e.g., 3–5 years, if a devoted program of investigation was undertaken. For example, Chandra [1992] was able to observe significant effects of supplemental vitamins on a variety of invasive parameters of immune function and infectious disease outcomes within a 12-month period in a cohort of community-dwelling elderly volunteers. A similar approach in generally healthy populations of children and adults could provide further insight into the levels of vitamin intake required for optimal immunity. However, problems regarding the statistical power of such studies can be foreseen in healthy young adults where the incidence of infectious disease episodes might be limited to just once or twice annually.

Substantiation of the potential value of vitamin intakes beyond recommended dietary allowances, as suggested, for example, by studies of vitamin A in children and vitamins B_6 and E in older adults, will require carefully conducted human studies with appropriate measures of assessment of immunity. Unfortunately, the number of well-controlled clinical trials is limited, in part due to the expense of such work. A number of factors must be considered in the design of studies intended to examine the role of vitamins in immunocompetence. The study population must be carefully characterized not only for age and gender but for comparable health and nutritional status, including the concurrent use of drugs and dietary supplements. The most rigorous trials will incorporate a double-blind, placebo-control design and be conducted for a sufficient duration to ensure that an effect is produced and endures. Also, trials should test at least several doses of the vitamin, preferably ranging from dietary through supra-dietary intakes to determine not only the potential for efficacy but safety as well. Importantly, due to the intra- and inter-subject variability of immune responses, especially with in vitro tests, protocols should include more than one sampling period. As noted above, both in vitro and in vivo measures of immune responsiveness are important to interpret the outcome of the study. The time required to complete extensive clinical trals such as these may exceed the 3- to 5-year duration estimated for relatively simple interventions of a single vitamin administered at a single dose with measurement of only a limited number of outcome variables.

4. How should our current knowledge be communicated to the consumer?

As indicated above, the number of carefully controlled clinical trials demonstrating an immunoenhancing effect of vitamin intake higher than generally recommended levels are limited [Blumberg, 1994]. This makes it difficult to evaluate completely the consistency and strength of putative beneficial actions and safety. Nonetheless, several recent studies, e.g. by Bogden et al. [1994], Chandra [1992] and Meydani et al. [1997], suggest good reason to pursue further research and consider better communicating the published information to healthcare providers, particularly concerning practical interventions available through dietary supplements. Some investigators already advocate stronger positions. For example, Chandra [1997] has stated: 'The era of nutrient supplements to promote health and reduce illness is here to stay. In selected groups such as the elderly, there is overwhelming evidence of immunologic enhancement following such an intervention.' Indeed, while it may be premature to recommend to the general public pharmacologic doses of specific vitamins to enhance immune function, steps might well be taken to ensure nutritional adequacy in populations at high risk for compromised immune function, such as poor children and the elderly, through multivitamin dietary supplements formulated with physiologic concentrations. Nonetheless, all consumers should know that nutrition is a critical determinant of immunocompetence and that diets which are generous in vitamin-rich fruits and vegetables contribute importantly to overall health and well-being.

References

Alexander M, Newmark H, Miller RG: Oral beta-carotene can increase the number of OKT4+ cells in human blood. Immunol Lett 1985;9:221–225.

Alpha-Tocopherol, Beta-Carotene Cancer Prevention Study Group: The effect of vitamin E and beta-carotene on the incidence of lung cancer and other cancers in male smokers. N Engl J Med 1994; 330:1029–1035.

Anderson R: Vitamins in the maintenance of optimal immune function and in the prevention of phagocyte-mediated tissue damage and carcinogenesis; in Walter P (ed): The Scientific Basis for Vitamin Intake in Human Nutrition. Basel, Karger, 1995, pp 66–74.

Anderson R: Mechanisms in vitamin-mediated anti-inflammatory and immunomodulatory activity. Bibl Nutr Dieta. Basel, Karger, 2000, vol 55, pp 135–147.

Beisel WR: The history of nutritional immunology: Introduction and overview. J Nutr 1992a;122:591–596.
Beisel WR: The history of nutritional immunology. J Nutr Immunol 1992b;1:5–40.
Bendich A: Immunology: Functions to assess nutrient requirements. J Nutr Immunol 1995;47–56.
Blumberg JB: Vitamins; in Forse RA (ed): Diet, Nutrition and Immunity. Boca Raton, CRC Press, 1994, pp 237–246.
Blumberg JB: Status and functional impact of nutrition in older adults; in Schneider EL, Rowe JW (eds): Handbook of the Biology of Aging. Orlando, Academic Press, 1996, pp 393–414.
Bogden JD, Bendich A, Kemp FW, Bruening KS, Skurnick JH, Denny T, Baker H, Louria DB: Daily micronutrient supplements enhance delayed hypersensitivity skin test responses in older people. Am J Clin Nutr 1994;60:437–447.
Chandra RK: Effect of vitamin and trace-element supplementation on immune responses and infection in elderly subjects. Lancet 1992;340:1124–1127.
Chandra RK: Graying of the immune system. JAMA 1997;277:1398–1399.
Cunningham-Rundles S: Nutrient Modulation of the Immune Response. New York, Dekker, 1993.
Gershwin ME, Beach RS, Hurley LS: Nutrition and Immunity. New York, Academic Press, 1985.
Hennekens CH, Buring JE, Manson JE, Stampfer M: Lack of effect of long-term supplementation with beta-carotene on the incidence of malignant neoplasms and cardiovascular disease. N Engl J Med 1996;334:1145–1149.
Hughes DA, Wright AJA, Finglas PM, Peerless ACJ, Bailey AL, Astley SB, Pinder AC, Southon S: The effect of beta-carotene supplementation on the immune function of blood monocytes from healthy male nonsmokers. J Lab Clin Med 1997;129:309–317.
Keusch GT, Wilson CS, Waksal SD: Nutrition, host defenses, and the lymphoid system. Arch Host Def Mech 1983;2:275–359.
Keusch GT, Farthing MJG: Nutrition and infection. Annu Rev Nutr 1986;6:131–154.
Meydani SN, Wu D, Santos MS, Hayek MG: Antioxidants and immune response in aged persons: Overview of present evidence. Am J Clin Nutr 1995;62:1462S–1476S.
Meydani SN, Meydani M, Blumberg JB, Leka LS, Siber G, Loszewski R, Thompson C, Pedrosa MC, Diamond RD, Stollar D: Vitamin E supplementation and in vivo immune response in healthy elderly subjects: A randomized controlled trial. JAMA 1997;277:1380–1386.
Mosmann TR, Sad S: The expanding universe of T-cell subsets: Th1, Th2 and more. Immunol Today 1996;17:138–146.
Omenn GS, Goodman GE, Thornquist MD: Effect of a combination of beta-carotene and vitamin A on lung cancer and cardiovascular disease. N Engl J Med 1996;334:1150–1155.
Santos MS, Meydani SN, Leka L, Wu D, Fotouhi N, Meydani M, Hennekens CH, Gaziano JM: Natural killer cell activity in elderly men is enhanced by beta-carotene supplementation. Am J Clin Nutr 1996;64:772–777.
Scrimshaw NS, Taylor CE, Gordon JE: Interaction of nutrition and infection. Am J Med Sci 1959;237: 367–403.

Prof J.B. Blumberg, USDA Human Nutrition Research Center on Aging,
Tufts University, 711 Washington Street, Boston, MA 02111-1524 (USA)
Tel. +1 617 556 3334, Fax +1 617 556 3295, E-Mail Blumberg@bnrc.tufts.edu

Walter P, Hornig D, Moser U (eds): Functions of Vitamins beyond Recommended Dietary Allowances. Bibl Nutr Dieta. Basel, Karger, 2001, No 55, pp 206–208

Emerging Scientific Evidence

Vitamin K and Bone Metabolism: Effects of Vitamins on Behaviour and Cognition

W. A. Rambeck[a], *H. B. Stähelin*[b]

[a] Lehrstuhl für Tierernährung, Ludwig-Maximillians-Universität, München, Deutschland;
[b] Geriatric University Clinic, Kantonspital, Basel, Switzerland

Vitamin K functions as a cofactor in the conversion of protein-bound glutamate residues into γ-carboxyglutamate (Gla). Initially, vitamin K was thought to be needed only for the synthesis of the four blood-clotting factors II, VII, IX and X. In recent years there is new interest in this vitamin because other functions have been discovered. Several proteins related to calcium homeostasis, for instance, are also synthesized in a vitamin K-dependent way. In bone, osteocalcin is an abundant Gla-containing protein, and although its function is not yet undestood completely, circulating osteocalcin serves as a valuable marker for osteoblastic bone formation. Vitamin K deficiency can easily be detected by measuring undercarboxylated osteocalcin (ucOC) in serum. A well-known risk group for vitamin K deficiency are newborns, who may develop the hemorrhagic disease of the newborn (HDN). Accumulating evidence shows that a mild form of vitamin K deficiency is also common in the elderly: Subjects with osteoporotic hip fractures had circulating vitamin K levels which were less than 30% of normal, and had elevated levels of ucOC. Supplementation of vitamin K led to normalization of ucOC, and to an increase of bone formation markers as well as to a reduction of urinary calcium loss.

The requirement of vitamin K for adults is around 1 μg/kg body weight per day, which is equivalent to about 10 g of spinach, and ensures optimal hemostasis. This amount was subsequently accepted as RDA value in the USA and in Great Britain. However, optimal glutamate carboxylation of bone Gla proteins may require higher vitamin K intakes. Clinical studies in which volunteers were supplemented with 1–10 mg/day suggest that the nutritional vitamin K intake should be equivalent to at least 100 g of spinach per day to meet the requirement of bone tissue.

Side effects of higher vitamin K supplementation are neither known from animal experiments nor from human high-dose supplementation. In Japan, e.g. 45 mg/day of vitamin K are given to postmenopausal women over several years. This dose is approximately 1,000 times the present RDA value. Some questions are still open. The interaction of higher vitamin K supplementation with oral anticoagulants, for instance, should be better understood. Also, clinical trials investigating the relation between the rate of postmenopausal bone loss and vitamin K should be performed. In two or three institutes, such trials have recently been started. Since both the availablility of endogenously produced vitamin K (in the colon) as well as the vitamin K uptake from food are low, supplementation of vitamin K is essential for babies, and should be considered for elderly people. This is especially true since recent investigations not only demonstrate positive effects of vitamin K on bone, but also a potential role for this vitamin in the prevention of atherosclerosis.

Increasing evidence links oxidative stress to neuronal damage, suggesting that antioxidants, particularly antioxidant vitamins, might have a protective effect. Observational epidemiological studies where high intake of β-carotene as well as other carotenoids, vitamin C and vitamin E correlate in healthy individuals with better cognitive performance compared to subjects with low intake support this hypothesis. However, not only oxidative stress to neurons, but other neurotoxic factors such as homocysteinemia and impaired metabolism of C-1 fragments in vitamin B_{12} and folic acid deficiency may be important. The regeneration of glutathione – which is in part dependent on vitamin B and antioxidants – essential for astrocytic and neuronal energy metabolism might affect cognitive performance. So far, epidemiological studies indicate less impairment in subjects with recommended intake compared to subjects with intake in the low range. With few exceptions, no reliable experimental human studies exist with intakes above RDAs. Two clinical trials with very high intake of vitamin E found also a favorable outcome in Parkinson's disease and Alzheimer's disease. However, part of the effect might be mediated by improving cerebral circulation, adding yet another mechanism to the possible interaction between vitamins, cognition and behavior. Antioxidants have been implicated in processes related to atherosclerosis, aging and selective neuronal damage, all of which may ultimately affect cognitive function and behavior. In understanding these mechanisms, the interaction of vitamins with genes will become very important. This approach may open new ways to define requirements (Azzi). The impact of this method on the concept of RDAs is at present not sufficiently clear. Nevertheless, it suggests e.g. that for vitamin E the target plasma concentration should be 40 µmol/l. At present, the database on the effect of vitamins on cognition and behavior is insufficient to recommend a general increase above RDAs. The recommendation for a high intake of fruit and vegetables should, however, be maintained and encouraged further. In order to advance knowledge, research in bioavailability of carotene, vitamins C and E, their kinetics and dynamics should be encouraged. In clinical and epidemiological intervention studies, optimal dosages as well as duration of exposure of vitamin E, carotene and vitamin C should be explored. In preventing cognitive impairment and behavioral disturbances, the benefit to individual and public health could be substantial and cost-effective.

Prof. W. A. Rambeck, Lehrstuhl für Tierernährung, Ludwig-Maximillians-Universität,
Veterinärstrasse 13, D–80539 München (Germany)
Tel. +49 8921 8032280

Author Index

Subject Index